CW01507056

Diverticulitis Diet Guide

A Detailed and Simple Guide with Easy and Delicious Recipes.

Author: Sophia Robinson

Legal Notice:
Copyright 2021 by Sophia Robinson - All rights reserved.

This document is geared towards providing exact and reliable information regarding the topic and issue covered. The publication is sold on the idea that the publisher is not required to render an accounting, officially permitted, or otherwise, qualified services. If advice is necessary, legal or professional, a practiced individual in the profession should be ordered.

From a Declaration of Principles which was accepted and approved equally by a Committee of the American Bar Association and a Committee of Publishers and Associations.

Legal Notes:
In no way is it legal to reproduce, duplicate, or transmit any part of this document by either electronic means or in printed format. Recording of this publication is strictly prohibited and any storage of this document is not allowed unless with written permission from the publisher. All rights reserved.

The information provided herein is stated to be truthful and consistent, in that any liability, in terms of inattention or otherwise, by any usage or abuse of any policies, processes, or directions contained within is the solitary and utter responsibility of the recipient reader. Under no circumstances will any legal responsibility or blame be held against the publisher for any reparation, damages, or monetary loss due to the information herein, either directly or indirectly. Respective authors own all copyrights not held by the publisher.

Disclaimer Notice:
The information herein is offered for informational purposes solely and is universal as so. The presentation of the information is without a contract or any type of guarantee assurance. Readers acknowledge that the author is not engaging in the rendering of legal, financial, medical or professional advice. Please consult a licensed professional before attempting any techniques outlined in this book.

By continuing with this book, readers agree that the author is under no circumstances responsible for any losses, indirect or direct, that are incurred as a result of the information presented in this document, including, but not limited to inaccuracies, omissions and errors.

The trademarks that are used are without any consent, and the publication of the trademark is without permission or backing by the trademark owner. All trademarks and brands within this book are for clarifying purposes only and are the owned by the owners themselves, not affiliated with this document.

TABLE OF CONTENTS

3

PHASE 2 RECIPES: Low Residue Meals

PHASE 3 RECIPES: High Fiber Meals ..136

What Exactly is Diverticulitis?

Diverticular Disease, also referred to as, Diverticulitis, is an illness that causes tiny, inflamed sac-like pouches form on your intestinal walls. These sacs protrude through the colon's outer walls creating pockets known as diverticula.

This disease can be considered a silent killer as it entirely possible for it to be present yet undetected if the symptoms are mild. The symptoms could be as mild as light diarrhea or even constipation which can be mistaken as normal. These symptoms would continue to worsen until it develops into your first flare.

As the disease progresses, it goes through various stages. Each stage creating more diverticula (the small pouches mentioned earlier) causing some patients to suffer from thousands of small sacs that grow in size. On the flip side, there are also many patients that only have a single small sac (known as a diverticulum) generally with a diameter of less than a centimeter, though the possibility exists of the sac multiplying or growing over time.

The Latest Science on Diverticulitis

Over the past few years there have been a number of studies into the causes, symptoms, and possible treatments for diverticulitis. In the past five years, more and more countries have issued guidelines on Diverticulitis D with differences regarding covered topics and recommendations including treatments. Presently, there is a lack of certainty on the impact of different drugs on patients who suffer from asymptomatic diverticulosis. A silver lining, however, is that throughout the years of research, limited indications have suggested that a progressive increase in dietary fiber aids in reducing the risk of developing Diverticulitis.

Age & Diverticulitis - Diverticulitis in The Younger Population

In the U.S., Diverticular disease is found in more than half of individuals beyond 60 years old. Around 10%-25% of individuals with Diverticular disease will encounter an irritation of a diverticulum, bringing about contamination (diverticulitis).

Why is this so?

The odds of contracting Diverticular disease increases with age. The sacs would already be of a decent size before the age of 40, and are found in more than 74% of individuals beyond 80 years old years in the U.S.

The strong mass of the colon becomes thicker with age, despite the fact that the reason for this thickening is unclear. It might mirror the expanding weights required by the colon to eliminate feces.

For instance, an eating routine low in fiber can prompt little, hard stools which are hard to pass and which require expanded weight to pass. The absence of fiber and little stools additionally may permit fragments of the colon to shut off from whatever is left of the colon when the colonic muscle in the portion contracts.

The pressure in these shut off fragments may turn out to be high since the expanded weight can't disperse to whatever remains of the colon. After some time, high weights in the colon push the internal intestinal coating outward (herniation) through frail zones in the strong dividers. These pockets or sacs that create are called Diverticular.

Absence of fiber in the eating diet has been thought to be the in all likelihood reason for Diverticular, and there is a decent connection among social orders far and wide between the measure of fiber in the eating diet and the prevalence of Diverticular. In any case, examines have not discovered comparative connections amongst fiber and Diverticular inside individual social orders. Numerous individuals with

Diverticular disease have unnecessary thickening of the solid mass of the colon where the Diverticular structure. The muscle additionally contracts all the more unequivocally. These irregularities of the muscle might contribute variables in the development of Diverticular. Microscopic examination of the edges of the Diverticular hint at irritation, and it has been proposed that aggravation might be essential for the arrangement of the Diverticular and not only the consequence of them

How do Doctors Diagnose A Patient with Diverticulosis?

Medicinal services suppliers regularly discover Diverticulosis amid a normal x beam or a colonoscopy, a test used to peer inside the rectum and whole colon to screen for colon malignancy or polyps or to assess the wellspring of rectal dying.

In view of side effects and seriousness of disease, a man might be assessed and analyzed by an essential consideration doctor, a crisis division doctor, a specialist, or a gastroenterologist—a specialist who works in digestive diseases.

The medicinal services supplier will get some information about the individual's wellbeing, indications, inside propensities, eating regimen, and drugs, and will perform a physical exam, which may incorporate a rectal exam. A rectal exam is performed in the social insurance supplier's office; anesthesia is not required. To perform the exam, the human services supplier requests that the individual twist around a table or lie on one side while holding the knees near the mid-section. The medicinal services supplier slides a gloved, greased up finger into the rectum. The exam is utilized to check for torment, dying, or a blockage in the digestive system.

The social insurance supplier may plan one or a greater amount of the accompanying tests:

- **Blood Tests**

A blood test includes drawing a man's blood at a medicinal services supplier's office, a business office, or a healing facility and sending the example to a lab for examination. The blood test can demonstrate the nearness of irritation or paleness—a condition in which red platelets are less or littler than ordinary, which keeps the body's cells from getting enough oxygen.

- **Colonoscopy**

The colonoscopy is performed at a healing facility or an outpatient focus by a gastroenterologist. Prior to the test, the individual's social insurance supplier will give composed entrails prep directions to take after at home. The individual may need to take after an unmistakable fluid eating routine for 1 to 3 days before the test.

The individual may likewise need to take intestinal medicines and bowel purges the night prior to the test. By and large, light anesthesia, and perhaps torment pharmaceutical, people groups unwind for the test.

The patient will lie on a table while the gastroenterologist embeds an adaptable tube into the rear-end. A little camera on the tube sends a video picture of the intestinal coating to a PC screen. The test can demonstrate Diverticulosis and Diverticular sickness.

Cramping or bloating may happen amid the main hour after the test. Driving is not allowed for 24 hours after the test to permit the anesthesia time to wear off. Prior to the arrangement, individuals ought to make arrangements for a ride home. Full recuperation is normal by the following day, and individuals ought to have the capacity to do a reversal to their ordinary eating routine.

- **Examining Your Lower GI (Gastrointestinal) Arrangement**

A lower GI arrangement is an x-beam exam that is utilized to take a gander at the digestive organ. The test is performed at a doctor's facility or an outpatient focus by an x-beam specialist, and the pictures are translated by a radiologist. Anesthesia is not required.

The medicinal services supplier may give composed inside prep guidelines to take after at home before the test. The individual might be requested that take after a reasonable fluid eating regimen for 1 to 3 days before the strategy. A diuretic or douche might be utilized before the test. A purgative is pharmaceutical that extricates stool and expands solid discharges.

A bowel purge includes flushing water or purgative into the rectum utilizing a unique squirt bottle. These drugs cause the runs, so the individual ought to remain nearby to a restroom amid the inside prep. For the test, the individual will lie on a table while the radiologist embeds an adaptable tube into the individual's rear-end.

The colon is loaded with barium; making indications of Diverticular illness appear the entire more plainly on x beams. For a few days, hints of barium in the digestive organ can make stools be white or light hued. Douches and rehashed defecations may bring about butt-centric soreness. A medicinal services supplier will give specific directions about eating and drinking after the test.

- **CT Scans (Mechanized tomography)**

A CT sweep of the colon is the most widely recognized test used to analyze Diverticular infection. CT filters utilize a mix of x beams and PC innovation to make three-dimensional (3–D) pictures. For a CT sweep, the individual might be given an answer for beverage and an infusion of an exceptional color, called contrast medium. CT checks require the individual to lie on a table that slides into a passage molded gadget where the x beams are taken.

The technique is performed in an outpatient focus or a doctor's facility by an x-beam expert, and the pictures are deciphered by a radiologist—a specialist who represents considerable authority in medicinal imaging. Anesthesia is not required. CT sweeps can distinguish Diverticulosis and affirm the analysis of diverticulitis.

Causes and Symptoms of Diverticulitis

Scientists have carried out intensive research over the years but have unfortunately not been able to hammer down a definite cause for diverticulitis. The one commonality among all their findings, however, was that a large number of the subjects who developed the diseases happened to be people who lacked sufficient fiber in the way they opted to eat and live their lives.

Despite the fact that no concrete evidence to a specific cause was found, there have been many theories that have surfaced throughout the years as to what the cause may be. One such theory that has grown in popularity believes that diverticulitis occurs as a result of pressure on the colon during constipation. It argues that straining when constipated causes the small diverticula to balloon from the intestinal wall and lodges between the muscle bundles from build up inside the colon.

This theory, of course, has never been proven but it is the most logical theory to date. It goes further to pair the disease with age as the mass of the colon thickens as we get older. Though the reasoning behind the specific aspect is still unclear, it is argued to be comparable to the expanding weights required to help our colon dispose of feces.

A large number of patients suffering from Diverticular disease experience unnecessary thickening of the solid mass of the colon that acts as the Diverticular structure. The muscle in this area also contracts all the more unequivocally. It has also been argued that these muscle irregularities may very well contribute to the development of Diverticular Disease.

Closer examination of the edges of the Diverticular structure in numerous studies has hinted at irritation and possible aggravation, which has also led some scientists to believe that this disturbance in the colon may not be a result of the disease but a determining factor of the arrangement of the diverticula.

The ugly truth is that any of these possible theories could potentially be true. Without diving into the science, itself, it is impossible to pinpoint which ones hit the nail on the head. What we can narrow down, however is how the presence of diverticular affects the human body. With that in mind, let's explore a few of the main symptoms experienced when a person contracts diverticulitis.

Symptoms of Diverticulitis

There are many diverticulitis patients that do not experience daily symptoms outside of a flare. This, as you can imagine, makes diagnosis in difficult outside of routine tests for general digestive issues. This isn't the reality for all patients; however, some experience warning signs or symptoms including:

Severe Constipation
Constipation can become so severe in diverticulitis patients that it prevents the passage of both gas and stool through the large intestine, and hence, a person is unable to pass the unwanted nitrogenous wastes out of the body.

Severe Pain in the Abdomen

Some may argue that abdominal pain is the most frequent symptom as over 95% of patients experience cramps in the left lower portion of the abdomen. These cramps can vary from person to person, but has been generally described as an achy, dull, or even sharp pain in some cases. At times, this pain may radiate to the lower back. The pain is sudden and severe in most cases, but it can also be mild in some cases.

Fever

Many patients experience a light fever in the early stages of diverticulitis and though it isn't a defining factor it does suggest the presence of an underlying infection. It is often associated with altered bowel habits, chills or both.

Diverticular Bleeding

Though bleeding isn't common, it does occur in some patients. On the off chance that you have bleeding, it can be serious. Luckily, the bleeding in some cases may also stop on its own without requiring any form of treatment. Be that as it may, if you begin to experience any form of bleeding form your rectum, regardless of the amount, you should see a medical professional immediately.

To discover the site of the bleeding and stop it, a specialist may play out a colonoscopy. Your specialist may likewise utilize an automated tomography (CT) check or an angiogram to discover the bleeding site. An angiogram is a unique sort of x-beam in which your specialist strings a dainty, adaptable tube through an extensive corridor, frequently from your crotch to the bleeding region.

Urinary Symptoms
Another symptom that is not as widely linked to diverticulitis is urinary tract issues. These can vary from a burning sensation during urination, frequent urination, and other urinary related issues due to the position of the bladder and colon in the body.

Nausea & Vomiting
Diverticulitis patients often suffer from indigestion related symptoms such nausea, vomiting and heart burn.

Diverticulitis when controlled often times doesn't severely affect your life outside of a flare. On the flip side, however, when the symptoms are left uncontrolled until it's too late, several more serious complications can pop up as a result. Including, but not limited to, intestinal perforation, fistula or abscess formation, peritonitis, bleeding and stricture (blockade).

These complications, however, are often rare and mainly in patients who already have a compromised or weak immune system, for example, those with previous underlying autoimmune or chronic illnesses such as AIDs, cancer, heart disease, and diabetes to name a few. Or patients who have been taking steroids for a long period.

When Should I Seek Medical Assistance?

Go to a crisis division instantly on the off chance that you have known Diverticular or past episodes of diverticulitis and you encounter any of the accompanying symptoms:

- Steady fever going with stomach torment
- Serious stomach torment
- Steady obstruction with stomach swelling or bloating
- Serious torment or different symptoms you beforehand experienced during a session with diverticulitis
- Serious vomiting

Understanding the 3 Stages of Diverticulitis and Adjustments Needed for Each Stage

The Diverticulitis diet is made up of three main stages:

- **Phase 1 – Clear Fluids:** Eating during an active flare-up

- **Phase 2 – Low Residue Meals:** eating while recovering from a flare, and

- **Phase 3 – High Fiber Meals:** preventing a flare in the future.

As with any other diet, you will need to listen to your body throughout each stage and make adjustments to the diet slowly as you add new foods while closely monitoring your symptoms.

Phase 1 - During a Flare: Clear Fluids Diet

While going through an active flare, your symptoms can become extreme. Due to this it's smart for you to give your bowel a period of rest. As you can imagine the best way to do this is by sticking to a clear fluid diet. This will aid in your recovery as your body may outright reject solid foods.

It is vital to note that the clear fluid stage of the diet is NOT intended to be a long-term diet. In fact, the general expectation is that you remain in this stage for no more than a couple of days.

WARNING:
Restricting yourself to a clear fluid diet for an excessive amount of time may cause you to feel light-headed, weak, hungry and fatigued. You can also experience muscle wasting, excessive weight loss, and depletion of vitamins and minerals.

This occurs due to the fact that it's incredibly difficult to meet the body's daily caloric requirements for fat, protein and carbohydrates through a clear fluid diet. The average person will need to provide their body with at least 200 grams of carbohydrates to have enough energy to go through the day. If you struggle with low blood sugar, diabetes, or other blood sugar challenges, you may want to monitor your blood sugar levels during this stage.

What to Eat & Avoid on The Clear Fluids Diet

What to Eat	What to Avoid
Clear, fat-free broth	
	All solid foods
Dairy – Free Coffee or tea (no creamer or milk)	
	Smoothies
Pedialyte	
	Peanut Butter
Boost clear or Boost juice	
	Fruit skins, Seeds or Pulp
Gelatin Pulp-free juice	
	Yogurt Based Drinks
Sports drinks	
	Milk & Milk Alternatives
Soda	
	All Condiments
Pulp-free fruit ice pops	

Phase 2 - After a Flare-Up: Low-Residue/Soft Diet

A low-residue (or low-fiber) diet acts as the reintroduction phase, after your flare-up symptoms have mostly passed but before your body is ready for high-fiber foods. "Residue"

What to Eat	What to Avoid
Coffee, tea; decaffeinated coffee; cereal beverage; carbonated beverage.	
Any tender meat, fish or fowl; eggs; cottage cheese; mild cheese; cream style peanut butter.	Fried; highly seasoned meats (such as cold cuts); strong cheese.
Butter; margarine; cream; vegetable oil; crisp bacon; avocado; gravy; cream sauce; mildly seasoned salad dressings.	Olives; nuts, highly seasoned salad dressings.
Milk and milk beverages; yogurt made with allowed fruits.	All remaining dairy products.
All juices, cooked or canned fruits: applesauce, apricots, cherries, peaches, pears, pineapple; raw fruit:	All other cooked fruits; all other fresh fruit; dried fruits.

banana and citrus fruit only without membrane.	
Cooked mild-flavored vegetables: asparagus, green or wax beans, beets, peas, carrots, spinach, mushrooms, pumpkin, tomato juice, squash.	All other cooked vegetables; all raw vegetables.
Broth; bouillon; cream or canned soups made with foods allowed.	All other soups.
Gelatin, sherbet; ice cream; custard; pudding; cake; cookies; pastry, Sugar; honey; jelly; candy.	Any with coconut, nuts or disallowed fruit, all others; any with coconut, nuts or disallowed fruit.

Phase 3 - Diverticulitis Flare: High-Fiber Foods

This final stage in the diverticulitis diet is the High Fiber diet. This stage is used to maintain a balanced diet while preventing a future flare. It is basically your general day to day eating routine, and generally takes up the majority of your diverticulitis eating plan.

It is important to note, however, that you do not want to jump directly from a significantly low fiber diet (such as a clear fluid diet) directly to a high fiber diet, as this will do more harm to your colon than good. It is always best to ease into any stage of the plan that requires in increase in your fiber intake. Aim to increase your fiber intake by 2 to 4 grams per week until you reach the recommended amount for your age and biology. Bear in mind that as you increase your fiber, you also need to increase your water intake to help move the fiber through your intestinal tract.

What to Eat	What to Avoid
Barley	
	All solid foods
Broccoli	
	Smoothies
Cauliflower	
	Peanut Butter
Berries (especially raspberries and blackberries)	
	Fruit skins, Seeds or Pulp
Brown Rice	

26

Raw Vegetables	
Cereal Flax Pears Chickpeas Lentils Chia Seeds	Refined White Rice or Flour products
Kiwi	
Fish (though not a high fiber protein)	Milk & Milk Alternatives
Beans	
Hemp Seeds Poultry (though not high fiber proteins) Wild Rice	More than 2 servings of Red Meat per Week
Avocados Crunchy Nut Butters Whole-grain pastas, bran cereal, bread and crackers	

Gut Microbiome and Diverticulitis

Bacteria and microorganisms are omnipresent: they live on the skin, in the nose, and the intestine. Our gastrointestinal system, particularly the large intestine, is home to far more diverse populations. From the scientific point of view, doctors describe the complexity of microorganisms that live in humans with the term microbiota.

In recent times, medicine has shown much interest in life within the intestine; some have called it a "forgotten organ." A person's alimentary canal is the most densely populated ecosystem on Earth. About one hundred trillion microbes (bacteria, viruses, fungi) roam on the surface of the substantially oxygen-free intestine. It is a huge number, unimaginable, written in numbers, it corresponds to 100,000,000,000,000 and is a thousand times greater than the number of stars that make up our galaxy.

If we put together all our intestinal microbes giving them the shape of an organ, this would weigh from 0.9 to 2.7 kg, compared to the brain weighing 1.2 kg. First, there was the talk of bacterial "flora" in the intestine. But this concept does not do justice to reality. The word flora is originated from the Latin, and it indicates the growth of plants on a portion of land, therefore something static.

Plants always remain in the same place. The concept of "bacterial flora" dates back to the period in which it was imagined that bacteria grew on the mucosa like grass on the earth and that the inside of the body was not touched. For this reason, we also talked about "bacterial carpet." Today we know that we are a dynamic whole and bacteria penetrate inside us, penetrating us.

They do not generate only in portions of the border. Everywhere, on and in our bodies, the surfaces, the passages between the inside and the outside are covered with biofilms of bacteria which in turn are formed by microbes that remain, comes and goes in a dynamic process. In the wake of the pioneering of the Human Genome Project, which has identified every human gene, scientists are now able to sequence large amounts of DNA very quickly and cheaply.

Now it is even possible to identify dead microbes expelled from the body in defecation because their DNA remains intact. We felt that our microbes were not important, but science is beginning to reveal a different story to us. A story in which human life is intertwined with that of our hitchhikers, in which microbes manage the body, and it is not possible for the human body to be healthy without them.

How many genes are needed to form a human being? From the hypotheses of the group of the most prepared people on the planet surely a higher number, compared to the number of genes of the mice, which as we knew had 23,000.

With its timid 21,000 genes, the human genome is not much larger than that of a worm. It is half that of the rice plant, and even the simple water flea with 31,000 genes outclasses it. Certainly, a complex and sophisticated body like the human body needs more proteins, and therefore more genes, than that of a worm.

But these 21,000 genes are not the only genes that govern our body. We do not live alone. Each of us is a superorganism. Our cells, although much larger in weight and volume, are outnumbered in numbers, in the proportion of ten to one, by the cells of the microbes that live in and above us. Altogether, the microbes that live on the human body contain 4.4 million genes: here is the microbiome, the collective genome of the microbiota.

The Human Microbiome Project (HMP), a consortium of 200 researchers from 80 US research institutions in 5 years, analyzed the genome of microbes living on the human body, the microbiome, to identify which species are present.

From this variety of microorganisms, about 70% is in the gastrointestinal tract with a concentration that increases exponentially in the fecal-oral direction. All this population can be divided into two large groups:

1. The autochthonous bacteria that start to colonize the digestive tract from birth and, after weaning, they turn into permanent, stable colonies. The quality and quantity of some particular strains can provide such constant "imprinting" that it can be used for individual identification with a precision higher than that of fingerprints!

2. The allochthones bacteria is found in our intestine only in a short form without forming stable colonies, and they are introduced with food when their number increases they cause

imbalances that from simple dysbiosis can reach even more serious diseases.

As we proceed inside the gastrointestinal system, the environmental conditions change, and this determines the variety of microbial species that settle at different levels. The bacteria colonize the segments of the intestinal tube where they find the most suitable conditions for their development: however, anatomy and physiology are essential in determining the quantity and quality of microorganisms. In general, traits, where the contractile movement of the intestine (peristalsis) is more contained, are welcome.

Among the factors that regulate the balance of the bacterial population is the pH, which is the acidity or basicity of the environment, oxygen, nutrients, and the presence of competitors. All the bacteria that live in the gastrointestinal tract are also found in the faeces whose composition reproduces the balance that has been established in recent stretches.
In inflammatory bowel diseases, and not only, instead of a functioning microbiome, there is also a disorder in the intestinal microbes, and the result is an excess or defect of metabolic products, genetic activations, and enzymes.

This condition is called "dysbiosis." The term originated from the Greek words dys for "wrong," "disturbed" and bios for "life" and the ending "-osi" for "condition," "state." A simple way to identify a dysbiosis is the control of the stool surfacing in the toilet (correct eubiosis) compared to a sinking (dysbiosis in progress).

Why Do Our Bodies Need Bacteria?

The intestinal bacteria produce substances that act on the brain through the intestinal mucosa and cover different ways: blood, immune, and nervous. They carry out an enormous metabolic job and constitute a precious ecosystem that, if intact, is very important for health and well-being.

"The microbiota can be seen as a metabolic" organ "tuned to our physiology." (Backhed, 2004) They play a vital role in the digestion, assimilation, and elimination of food. Without bacteria it would be impossible to digest certain types of fiber properly. They feed and digest them for us, and in doing so, they also produce some nutrients we need.

Depending on the diet, the bacteria release a particular amount of active metabolic substances. The vitamins belong to these. Certain Bifidus and Escherichia Coli strains produce, as it was discovered in 1983, vitamins of the B group: B1, B2, B3 and their nicotinamide derivatives, B5, B6, B12, folic acid, biotin and vitamin K necessary for blood coagulation.

For their metabolism, for example, nerve cells need vitamin B12 and folic acid, both of which are supplied by food through the action of intestinal bacteria. Even a minimal deficiency of these trace elements can cause an insufficient supply to the nerves which have repercussions in the form of nervous weakness in the belly-brain-belly agreement.

The intestinal bacteria also perform a detoxifying function, neutralizing, for example, some substances that are harmful to our body, such as ammonia. The unhealthy microbiota developed, increases the levels of pro-inflammatory cytokines, such as IL-6 and IL-8 and lipopolysaccharide (LPS), which cause intestinal inflammation and permeability of the walls.

Furthermore, these inflammatory molecules contribute to the metabolic dysfunction with the altered metabolism of bile acid, the production of short-chain fatty acids, the secretion of the intestinal hormone, and the circulation of branched-chain amino acids. The most important role bacteria play in the reabsorption of bile acids. Bile is composed of bile salts, the bilirubin dye, cholesterol, and phospholipids. These are important for bile stabilization.

If the bile is salty, bilirubin or cholesterol crystallize, gallstones form, based on their relationship with phospholipids. Bile is formed in liver cells and the gall bladder and from there, depending on food intake, released into the small intestine. Bile also contains several enzymes and substances that the liver has filtered to purify the body.

If the intestine is not healthy, it can leave the liver with a more significant number of toxic substances through the bile to detoxify, then brought back into the intestine, through which they should be eliminated. If the microbiome is in good shape here, the intestinal bacteria carry out the steps necessary for detoxification; otherwise, they may be reabsorbed and returned to the liver.

Great attention was paid to the possible role of short chain fatty acids (SCFA acronym for Short Chain Fatty Acids) such as butyrate, propionate, and acetate since

SCFA are the main product of the digestive action of intestinal microbiota. It has been reported that SCFAs affect host metabolism through various parallel pathways associated with protein-coupled receptors, and these receptors are active in neuroendocrine cells in the intestine and can, therefore, influence brain signaling.

The more a disturbance persists in the intestinal mucosa, in the form of a reduction in the number of microbes, a modified composition, a lack of mucosa, inflammation, immune reactions and the higher the probability that the cells of the intestinal epithelium do what they want.

For nerve cells to at least be able to transmit impulses to other cells, communication, a compatible instrument is necessary for everyone. These are nerve messengers, neurotransmitters. Small molecules that are transported by a nerve cell in the space of the next one. Serotonin is one of the most vital neurotransmitters, and it is found mainly in the intestine. Its effects on the body affect all central, and vital areas: like the heart and circulation of blood coagulation, or regulation of eye pressure. It transmits mucosal stimuli to the tissues in the gastrointestinal tract, and as a result of this, the movements of the organs are coordinated.

Also, it occurs directly or indirectly, in almost all the functions of the central nervous system and of the enteric ones: the serotonin rule perception, sensitivity and temperature, tiredness and pain, stimulus development, hormonal production, and sexual behavior.

If there is enough serotonin in the body, the human being is balanced, if the serotonin is lacking, moods appear as prostration and killing, up to depression, dissatisfaction, irritability, fear, and aggressive behavior. It also performs protective functions and increases the barrier effect: increased production of mucin and zoludin is a component of the tight junctions (the tight junctions that allow the intestinal epithelium to act as a protective barrier towards the inside of the body).

Finally, the intestinal microbiota is essential for our immune system. About 70-80% of the body's immune cells are located in the intestine. The microbiota stimulates the maturation of the immune system and has a "barrier effect" against potential aggressors. The "good" bacteria (saprophytes or commensals) attach themselves to the intestinal wall and occupy the space, thus preventing the establishment of harmful bacteria.

Bacteria make the nerves grow or prevent its growth, and they make the connections grow or prevent them, inhibit, favor, or regulate. Bacteria determine brain activity, the values of blood and tissues of neurotransmitters, hormones, and hematocytes, as well as development and inflammation and vegetative reactions, depend on them. Intestinal bacteria is the part that accompanies us throughout our lives, and the brain development of our ability to feel, to behave and even to think, without them, we will not be a whole human being.

Some microorganisms can produce a neurotransmitter, gamma-aminobutyric acid. This substance, abbreviated as GABA, is one of the most abundant signaling molecules in the nervous system, which keeps the emotional part of our brain, the limbic system, under control. But it would be possible to use this knowledge to treat anxiety disorders with GABA-producing microbes in the form of probiotics.

So how does this all tie in with Diverticulitis?

When diverticulitis, like other digestive illnesses are caused by excessive proliferation of harmful bacteria or poor differentiation of bacterial strains, the microbiota will produce harmful effects on the rest of the body and then to the brain. The "bad" bacteria will produce toxic substances, called "neurotoxins," for the nervous system.

These neurotoxins will eventually alter mental functions, generating stress, anxiety, and even psychiatric or neurodegenerative diseases. An imbalance in the intestinal microbiota will have the effect of depleting or over-stimulating the immune system. The harmful bacteria that prevail over those beneficial alters of the intestinal wall can make it porous, allowing the passage of macromolecules and foreign toxins into the blood.

These intruders cause the immediate reaction of intestinal immune cells, which will alert the entire immune system, releasing inflammatory molecules and stress hormones. In this way, the harmful intestinal bacteria can start a state of chronic inflammation, with negative effects on the brain and our mental health.

How to Improve Gut Flora

The human body is comprised of over 40 trillion bacteria that has multiple purposes, a number which reside in your intestines. The good bacteria as a collective are referred to as the gut microbiota or gut flora, and they play an extremely vital part in maintaining your overall health. The bad bacteria that form, on the other hand, contributes to many different diseases.

Due to this it is vital that you take care of your gut to ensure that most the bacteria residing in your body is good bacteria. As you may have already guessed, the food you consume plays a significant role in the type of bacteria that grow inside you.

Let's explore a few simple ways you can improve your gut flora:

Maintaining Bacterial Balance

One of the symptoms that are very common in diverticulitis patients is the intestinal bacterial overgrowth. That is too much development of harmful bacteria which leads to inflammation and damage to the entire system and makes all digestion less effective. Rifaximin is a drug that has been shown to affect this issue in a positive way by returning the bacterial balance to a more normal level. There are also simple foods that will do this as well, including some specialty yogurts.

Eat regularly

It is important to develop a normal eating schedule each day. It is believed that eating all of your snacks and meals at the same time each day will allow for your digestive system and colon to work in a more regular fashion and that will keep your colon in great shape and avoid the development of Diverticular disease.

Make a goal to have your main three meals at about the same time each day along with any snacks. Most people are creatures of habit and this can become easy to do.

Lean Meats

If you are going to consume meats, ensure that they are lean meats. Meats that have an excess of fatty tissue in them are not healthy for the digestion and they can introduce too much of the unhealthy kinds of bacteria in the colon, a perceived cause of diverticulitis. Some smart meats to eat are skinless poultry, pork loin and select lean cuts of steak.

Gain an Understanding of Fiber and How It Affects Your Gut

Doctors that specialized in digestive tract illnesses have looked at what most people eat as a daily part of their diet and found that it is lacking in many of the essential nutrients that people should be eating for excellent digestive health.

One of these ingredients is a diet that is much higher in fiber than is previously prescribed. One of the major contributors to the development of diverticulitis is that a person has difficulty in passing waste out of the colon through the rectum.

A diet high in fiber will make this much easier and alleviate much of the problem. After the muscles in a person's colon spend years straining to perform their function due to a diet that is low in fiber there is a development of this issue. Particularly in the United States this can be seen. Doctors start to realize that the colon is becoming a bit stretched which makes it even more difficult to pass excrement from the body and the stool needs to be even bulkier to be moved out without difficulty.

There was a study done by the Journal of Nutrition that observed nearly 45,000 health professionals participating in a long-term study. They learned that when a person ate a diet that was high in fiber, they lowered the risk of contracting Diverticular disease by somewhere in the neighborhood of 40%.

A high fiber diet presents a lot of other benefits as well. It fills your stomach easily and suppresses your appetite with can have a major assist in losing weight. Losing weight can help fight against developing Diverticular disease indirectly. Diverticular disease is much more likely to put a woman in the hospital if she is overweight or inactive. This is according to a study that was published in the American Journal of Gastroenterology.

It is recommended currently that 25 grams of fiber should be consumed by women each and every day. While men should eat even more fiber, being advised to try to consume about 38 grams of fiber in the daily diet. Even with these warnings the average American eats about 15 grams of fiber a woefully low portion. One of the best ways to augment your lack of fiber is to include foods that are high in fiber at every meal and also for snacks throughout the day.

Great sources of fiber for your diet include whole grains, oatmeal whole wheat bread, and barley. There are also some other great foods that you can dig into like lentils, fruits, vegetables and beans to give your diet a kick. One of the best snacking foods for a fiber input into your diet is to eat plenty of dried fruits which are a terrific source of fiber.

This type of eating plan is referred to as a whole foods diet because it includes a lot of foods that are not processed and treated with chemicals like white rice and white bread. Both of these are going to help cause diverticulitis rather than cure it. Eliminating the food that is bad for you is just as important as adding the food that is good for the body.

There are two types of fiber to consider soluble and insoluble. They are both an important part of a healthy diet but for different reasons. The insoluble fiber that is found in vegetable peels of fruit and seeds will add bulk to the stool in the colon and make it easier to pass reducing the wearing strain on the muscle. Soluble fiber is the other kind that a body needs, and it comes from foods like oatmeal, barley, and many fresh fruits like apples. This adds to the moisture located in the stool and that makes it easier to pass through the colon and reduces the strain.

The recommended intake of fiber is generally:
- Women age 19 to 50 = 25 grams per day
- Women age 50+ = 21 grams per day
- Men age 19 to 50 = 38 grams per day

- Men age 50+ = 30 grams per day

Please contact your doctor to confirm that these values are okay for your specific scenario.

Drink More Fluids

Many overlook the importance of staying hydrated, but this tip may be the most effective in maintaining gut health. Drinking more fluids can help a high fiber diet be moved even easier through the digestive process with fewer chances of obstructions developing. Keeping the fluid intake into a normal level is all that is needed. There doesn't seem to be much of a benefit for drinking excessive liquids during the day. Look to drink as many non-calorie beverages as you can with your diet each day that means no limits to water or tea.

The recommended water intake is generally:
- Men age 19+ = 12 cups (about 3 liters) per day
- Women age 19+ = 9 cups (about 2 liters) per day

Please contact your doctor to confirm that these values are okay for your specific scenario.

Available Diverticulitis Treatments

A person suffering from diverticulitis may be able to find some significant relief by taking probiotic supplements. In combination with other treatments the probiotic nutrients can give a person a whole new lease on life. There are some great food choices that already include probiotics in them for example eating foods with kefir, kimchi or kombucha in them will naturally help reduce the effects of diverticulitis.

Adding a supplement like Prescript Assist or VSL#3 is not a bad idea no matter where your health is currently at because it will improve your digestion and allow you to feel healthier each day.

Probiotics

It is important to make sure probiotics are in your diet. Probiotics will add healthy bacteria to the digestive system and make the colon work smoother and more efficiently which will allow for less development of Diverticular disease. Probiotics enhance the ability of the body to take the nutrients from food, breakdown lactose and even help improve the immune system of the body. Low fat yogurt or kefirs are a great source of probiotics for people to consume in order to avoid Diverticular disease.

Prebiotics are another option when it comes to correcting the level of good/bad bacteria in the digestive system. These are substances that are known to develop and nurture the growth and development of the positive forms of bacteria that will keep you healthy and manage your wellbeing.

This is exactly what a person is looking for when they need to restore a healthy bacterial balance. One great probiotic is fructose-oligosaccharide powder but consult a doctor or doctor to learn about more prebiotics that can help in solving a poor bacterial balance and help to stop diverticulitis before it begins.

Stay away for foods high in fat. It is no secret that foods that are high in fat tend to slow down the digestion process and can lead to episodes of constipation. This is not healthy for the colon because it causes undue stress on the muscles and can cause long term damage to them. It is also much easier to maintain a healthy weight if the foods that are high in fat are avoided.

Approved Diverticulitis Foods

It is important to remember that having diverticulitis does not mean that there are going to be any symptoms visible for a person to observe. Many live blissfully unaware of their condition until they have an attack and then that painful uncomfortable situation will need to be treated by a medical professional. One of the simple cures is with antibiotics but there are more serious cases that need to be handled with surgery.

Again, we know that if you are suffering from diverticulitis, a liquid diet may be prescribed by your doctor as being included in your treatment. This will give the colon a chance to heal and recover without having to perform the task that it was designed for.

This type of liquid diet should include tea, water, ice pops, broth and fruit juices. Very slowly the patient can start to readd solid foods back in your diet. However, they really need to stop neglecting the fiber at this point and start to eat high fiber foods. Because of the medical condition the colon might have difficulty at first passing high fiber foods very well so your doctor will most likely prescribe foods that are lower in fiber to begin with.

These include eggs, fish, poultry and all dairy products as well. Remember the more fiber that is present in the diet the more bulk there will be in the stool and that will reduce the pressure on the colon to perform its job.

There have been studies done that demonstrate quite clearly that foods that are rich in fiber helps to curve the onset of diverticulitis and the flares it brings to the table. Again, it is urged that you be sure to consume at least 25 grams of fiber daily.

Phases/Stages of the Diverticulitis Diet & How To Eat During Each Phase

There are three main phases of the Diverticulitis diet: eating during an active flare-up, eating while recovering from a flare, and preventing a flare in the future. As with any other diet, you will need to listen to your body throughout each stage and adjust the diet slowly as you add new foods while closely monitoring your symptoms.

Phase 1: Clear Fluids (During A Flare)

While going through an active flare, your symptoms can become extreme. Due to this it's smart for you to give your bowel a period of rest. As you can imagine the best way to do this is by sticking to a clear fluid diet. This will aid in your recovery as your body may outright reject solid foods.

It is vital to note that the clear fluid stage of the diet is NOT intended to be a long-term diet. In fact, the general expectation is that you remain in this stage for no more than a couple of days.

Please Note:
Restricting yourself to a clear fluid diet for an excessive amount of time may cause you to feel light-headed, weak, hungry, and fatigued. You can also experience muscle wasting, excessive weight loss, and depletion of vitamins and minerals.

This occurs due to the fact that it's incredibly difficult to meet the body's daily caloric requirements for fat, protein, and carbohydrates through a clear fluid diet. The average person will need to provide their body with at least 200 grams of carbohydrates to have enough energy to go through the day. If you struggle with low blood sugar, diabetes, or other blood sugar challenges, you may want to monitor your blood sugar levels during this stage.

As the name implies, this phase is composed of clear liquids. These include green tea, fresh fruit juice, clear broth, and gelatin dessert. The clear liquid diet provides the body with salt, liquids, and enough nutrients to function temporarily, **generally for a few days,** until you can eat normal food.

Phase 2: Low-Residue/Low Fiber Diet (Immediately After A Controlled Flare)

A low-residue (or low-fiber) diet acts as the reintroduction phase, after your flare-up symptoms have mostly passed but before your body is ready for high-fiber or high residue foods.

Phase 3: High Fiber Meals (Daily Life/ Preventing Future Flares)

This final stage in the diverticulitis diet is the High Fiber diet. This stage is used to maintain a balanced diet while preventing a future flare. It is basically your general day to day eating routine, and generally takes up the majority of your diverticulitis eating plan.

It is important to note, however, that you do not want to jump directly from a significantly low fiber diet (such as a clear fluid diet) directly to a high fiber diet, as this will do more harm to your colon than good. It is always best to ease into any stage of the plan that requires an increase in your fiber intake.

Aim to increase your fiber intake by 2 to 4 grams per week until you reach the recommended amount for your age and biology. Bear in mind that as you increase your fiber, you also need to increase your water intake to help move the fiber through your intestinal tract.

Essential Shopping List

Fruits
- ☐ Apple Sauce
- ☐ Apples
- ☐ Apricots
- ☐ Bananas
- ☐ Dates
- ☐ Mangoes
- ☐ Oranges
- ☐ Peaches
- ☐ Prunes

Juices
- ☐ Apple Juice
- ☐ Lemon Juice
- ☐ Lime Juice
- ☐ Orange Juice
- ☐ Cranberry Juice

Vegetables
- ☐ Alfalfa Sprouts
- ☐ Artichoke Hearts
- ☐ Asparagus
- ☐ Avocados
- ☐ Black Olives
- ☐ Broccoli
- ☐ Butternut Squash
- ☐ Cabbage
- ☐ Carrots
- ☐ Cauliflower
- ☐ Celery
- ☐ Eggplants
- ☐ Garlic
- ☐ Green Bell Peppers (seedless)
- ☐ Green Olives
- ☐ Green Onions
- ☐ Leeks
- ☐ Mushrooms
- ☐ Lettuce
- ☐ Olives
- ☐ Onions
- ☐ Peas (frozen, cooked)
- ☐ Pimento
- ☐ Red Bell Peppers (seedless)
- ☐ Russet Potatoes
- ☐ Shallots
- ☐ Spinach
- ☐ Sugar Snap Peas
- ☐ Summer Squash
- ☐ Yellow Peppers (seedless)
- ☐ Tomatoes (seedless)
- ☐ Water chestnuts
- ☐ Zucchini
- ☐ Sweet Yams

Beans & Peas
- ☐ Black Beans
- ☐ Butter Beans
- ☐ Cannellini Beans
- ☐ Garbanzo Beans
- ☐ Canned Kidney Beans
- ☐ Lentils
- ☐ Canned Lima Beans
- ☐ Canned Navy Beans
- ☐ Canned Red Beans

Grains, Breads & Other Starches
- ☐ All Bran Cereal
- ☐ Barley
- ☐ Brown Rice
- ☐ Fiber One Cereal
- ☐ Long Grain Rice
- ☐ Oat Bran
- ☐ Rolled Oats
- ☐ Whole Wheat Tortellini
- ☐ Whole Wheat Flour
- ☐ Whole Wheat Pasta
- ☐ Whole Wheat Pita
- ☐ Whole Wheat Tortillas
- ☐ Whole Wheat Bread

Meats
- ☐ Crab Meat, Cooked
- ☐ Ground Chicken, Lean
- ☐ Ground Turkey, Lean
- ☐ Lean Ham
- ☐ Shrimp, large, peeled
- ☐ Canned Tuna Fish, in water
- ☐ Turkey Breast
- ☐ Chicken Breast

Dairy
- ☐ Cheddar Cheese (low fat)
- ☐ Cottage Cheese (low fat)
- ☐ Cream Cheese (low fat)
- ☐ Feta Cheese
- ☐ Monterrey Jack Cheese (low fat)
- ☐ Parmesan Cheese
- ☐ Eggs
- ☐ Half and half cream

- Milk, low fat
- Yogurt, low fat

Spices, Herbs & Oils
- Baking Powder
- Basil (fresh or dried)
- Canola Oil
- Cilantro (fresh)
- Cinnamon powder
- Cumin
- Curry Powder
- Dill, (fresh or dried)
- Italian Seasoning
- Nutmeg
- Olive Oil
- Oregano, (fresh and dried)
- Parsley, Italian (fresh)
- Sage (fresh)
- Tarragon (fresh)
- Thyme (fresh and dried)
- Vanilla

Condiments
- Vegetable Stock
- Chicken Stock
- Coconut Milk

- Dijon Mustard
- Honey
- Light Ranch Dressing
- Maple Syrup
- Mayonnaise, low fat
- Red Wine Vinegar
- Rice Vinegar
- Soy Sauce
- Sweet Pickle Relish
- Tarragon Vinegar
- Tomato Paste
- Tomato Sauce
- Tomato Puree
- Canned Tomato, diced, seedless

List of Foods to Avoid

Patients with diverticulitis are often urged to exercise caution when consuming seeds or anything with seeds (i.e., tomatoes, melons, berries, etc.). Small foods particles such as seeds are theorized to potentially be able to get logged in the diverticulum and cause inflammation.

Although there hasn't been any scientific evidence to date that would confirm this belief, I will be including seeds and nuts in our Foods to Avoid list and omit them from my recipes.

Be sure to consult your doctor to see whether you would be permitted to including them in your diet.

There are several reasons why certain foods should be avoided during the acute (symptomatic) phase of diverticulitis. Some of these reasons include:

- Increase the bulk of the stool: Some of these foods are high in fiber and, therefore, contribute to the consistency and bulk of the stool. In many cases, as a person already suffers from severe constipation, increased intake of such foods will only make it harder to defecate and will eventually result in more abdominal discomfort.

- Some of these foods can get caught in the pouches called diverticula.

51

- Take longer time for digestion: Some of these foods take a longer time to digest. As the digestive system is already sore (inflamed), and under abnormally high-pressure during diverticulitis, more of such foods will only create more complications, and as a result, the stomach and intestines would not get the "rest" they need the most during diverticulitis.

- Produce flatulence and bloating: Intestinal gas and bloating are common side effects of a high fiber diet. Presence of such symptoms will increase the risk of more complications in diverticulitis attack.

Vegetables with Small Particles or Seeds

- Cucumber (only English is acceptable)
- Green Peppers (Acceptable if seeds are removed)
- Tomato (Acceptable if seeds are removed)
- Chili Peppers
- Corn

Seeds & Nuts

- Avoid all types

Sweets with Small Particles or Seeds

- Nutty Candy
- Fruit Jam with Seeds
- Nutty Desserts
- Raisins with Seeds

Fruits with Small Particles or Seeds

- Blackberries
- Blueberries
- Coconut (dried)
- Whole Cranberries (Cranberry Relish)
- Figs
- Grapes with seeds
- Kiwi
- Pomegranates
- Raspberries
- Strawberries
- Watermelon (Acceptable if seedless)

Starches (Refined)

- Bread or rolls with nuts/seeds
- Popcorn
- Wild Rice

53

How to Deal with Attacks

Patients may have various scenes of Diverticular disease or diverticulitis and might be hard to recognize the two. Milder scenes of torment might be dealt with at home with bed rest, prescriptions for torment and fit, and an unmistakable fluid diet. Patients ought to take their temperature as often as possible and push on their lower left guts where most Diverticular are found.

At the principal indication of fever or expanding delicacy - indications of aggravation - a specialist ought to be counseled instantly for a conceivable visit to his office and/or the start of anti-infection agents; there is nothing as profitable as a physical examination by the specialist to settle on choices about further treatment or hospitalization.

How to Deal with Mild to Medium Symptoms

Most patients with Diverticulosis have negligible or no symptoms, and don't require a particular treatment. A typical fiber diet is fitting to counteract blockage and maybe keep the arrangement of more Diverticular.

Patients with gentle symptoms of stomach pain because of strong fit in the range of the Diverticular may profit by hostile to uncontrollable medications, for example:

- Hyoscyamine (Levsin)
- Phenobarbital (Donnatal)
- Chlordiazepoxide (Librax)
- Dicyclomine (Bentyl)
- Scopolamine
- Atropine

At the point when diverticulitis happens, anti-toxins for the most part are required. Oral anti-infection agents are adequate when symptoms are gentle.

A few cases of normally recommended anti-microbials include:

- Flagyl (metronidazole)
- Cipro (Ciprofloxacin)
- Keflex (Cephalexin)
- Vibramycin (doxycycline)

What are different medications for diverticulitis?

Fluid or low fiber foods are informed during intense attacks with respect to diverticulitis. This is done to decrease the measure of material that goes through the colon, which in any event hypothetically, may irritate the diverticulitis. In extreme diverticulitis, where patients suffer from intense pain and high fever, the patients are often hospitalized to be treated with intravenous anti-infection agents. Surgery is required for patients with steady entrails obstacle, bleeding, or sore not reacting to antibiotics.

55

How to Deal with Strong Symptoms

Diverticulitis that does not react to restorative treatment requires surgical mediation. Surgery normally includes drainage of any collections of discharge and resection (surgical evacuation) of the portion of the colon containing the Diverticular, as a rule the sigmoid colon. Surgical expulsion of the bleeding diverticulum likewise is important for those with determined bleeding. In patients requiring surgery to stop industrious bleeding, it is important to decide precisely where the bleeding is originating from keeping in mind the end goal to direct the specialist.

Now and then, Diverticular can disintegrate into the nearby urinary bladder, creating serious intermittent pee contamination and entry of gas amid pee. This circumstance additionally requires surgery.

Now and then, surgery might be proposed for patients with regular, repetitive attacks of diverticulitis prompting different courses of anti-toxins, hospitalizations, and days lost from work. During surgery, the objective is to evacuate all, or all, of the colon containing Diverticular so as to anticipate future occurrences of diverticulitis.

How to Deal with Abdominal Pain

Chronic abdominal pain can be a really challenging symptom for many of us, particularly when it sticks around for a really long time. pain is a challenge for not only kids and teenagers, but also for the parents. This section was intended to attempt to give you a clearer understanding as to why we have abdominal pains and what we can do about it.

What is the purpose of pain in the first place if you think about it. Pain serves to protect us from harm, for example, if you touch a hot pan on the stove you get a painful sensation in your hand that lets you know that you need to move your hand away quickly to avoid getting burned. If we didn't have pain signals we wouldn't know to move our hand away from the hot pan.

In this example, we can see that the pain signals are serving a very specific purpose; to keep us out of harm's way. Unfortunately, pain signals can go haywire sometimes. With acute pain, like breaking your arm for example, we experience pain initially but then heal over time and return back to normal functioning. With chronic pain, however, this pain goes on for much longer than expected our pain alarms have gone haywire.

Did you know you have two brains? Yes! You have the one in your skull, but you also have one in your gut. With chronic abdominal pain, we have pain signals going back and forth between our gut and our brain. In many cases our gut brain may be hypersensitive to

various sensations which causes it to send a pain alarm to the brain in our skull. The gut brain may be yelling, "Emergency! Emergency!" to the skull brain when in
reality there is no danger at all.

The longer chronic abdominal pain lasts, the stronger the connection between the gut brain and skull brain becomes. We know that there is a very strong connection between the gut brain and the skull brain.

With chronic abdominal pains, there's also often a nerve problem. The nerves and our guts may be overly sensitive to stimulation. In addition, many parts of our lives can impact pain including:
- sleep
- diet
- exercise
- family
- relationships
- social functioning
- and even school

When things aren't going well with pain it is very common to catastrophize pain and think that things will never get better. So, what do we do about it?

The first step in treating chronic abdominal pain is understanding how it works. Through treatment, using a cognitive behavioral approach, we can start turning
down those pain alarms being sent from your gut brain to your skull brain just like turning down the volume on a radio.

Dietary Tips for Abdominal Pain

Outside of CBT there are also small dietary changes that you can implement to assist with abdominal pains in the short term. These include using:

- **Turmeric:**

Turmeric can be dated back to thousands of years as being used as a treatment for gut health and abdominal pains in both Indian and Chinese medicine. At the time, they weren't even sure why it worked. What was clear, was that it had been extremely effective. Today science confirms that this ancient therapy works and is discovering the secrets behind its success.

Take it slow when adding turmeric, and especially curcumin, supplements. Too much when your microbiome isn't use to it, or the wrong kind, can cause stomach irritation and mild diarrhea. The best way to supplement turmeric is as an ingredient in cooked food, especially one containing fat and pepper.

A very good way of doing this is by using "Turmeric Paste". This makes mixing it to any food or a warm drink very easy. Turmeric paste has been shown in scientific research studies to be 2,000 times more effective than "raw" turmeric. Not everyone will want to make their own paste (though it is pretty easy to do, and I think it is worth it), so try to cook with it (it has a very mild flavor). Raw turmeric and curcumin can be harsh to an already sensitive gut, so start at about half the bottle suggestion.

The best way to take Turmeric is as turmeric paste or cooked in food that contains a fat and black pepper.

Turmeric paste can be used in kefir, homemade yogurt, smoothies, soups, stews, casseroles, curry dishes, etc. You can even coat baked chicken with it before cooking to give up some color.

When adding turmeric or curcumin to your diet or supplements you need to make sure it is the most bioavailable form possible. Otherwise, it won't be helping you nearly as much, and it may even cause some intestinal discomfort.

- **Zinc:**

Zinc carnosine is a very valuable supplement for treating gut permeabilities like leaky gut and for healing the intestinal wall, both of which can contribute to abdominal pains.

The mere fact that Zinc is so heavily involved in enzymatic functions makes it very important for gut health. There are dozens of enzymes required for digestion, intimal tight junctions, etc.

When first starting, consume up to 40mg of zinc per day (as Zinc Carnosine) for the first 6 months. Maintenance - 8-16mg per day

- **l-Glutamine:**

This is a natural amino acid that is very useful for healing your stomach and small intestine. It is very helpful at healing the lining of the gut and permeable gut. Glutamine is the most popularly prescribed ulcer medication in Asia. It is also often used to treat Crohn's and other forms of IBD (Inflammatory bowel disease).

Many people have reported feeling some better within in a few days, especially when consuming bone broths as well. They often report greater energy and less fatigue. Be sure not to subject l-glutamine to high heat; if you use this as part of your smoothie using a high-speed blender make sure it includes ice.

If you feel that you have become anxious, or any anxiety has become worse, since starting glutamine you will need to stop taking it as a supplement. Women who are pregnant or trying to conceive should not supplement l-glutamine out of an abundance of caution.

Glutamine has been wrongly implicated as an excitotoxin, often confused with l-glutamate. There are some reports that l-glutamine might convert to the neuroexcitatory amino acid "l-glutamate", which can over excite brain neurons. There is also evidence to the contrary, and evidence that even if true it would not be any worse than the food ingredient MSG. But, better to be safe.

The amino acid Glutamine is a normal, and large, part of our diets. You would have to be a vegan to even start to avoid it, even then it would be difficult. Glutamine is converted to Glutamate as the body needs it. Glutamate is an excitotoxin, but small amounts of it are required in the brain, thus the reason why we have the ability to convert glutamine to glutamate. Glutamine is not an endotoxin! It is what the small intestine uses to heal itself; it is also required for life.

Using extra glutamine to help heal the gut is perfectly fine. What you want to avoid is ALL forms of MSG (a glutamate) and it goes by many names.

But because there is controversy, I would recommend that pregnant women, or people with a history of: liver disease, strokes, neurological disorders or multiple sclerosis, not supplement l-glutamine outside of their diets without first consulting their MD. Everyone else should probably not supplement l-glutamine for more than 3 months without taking a 2 month break. This last provision may not apply to athletes taking it before a workout as the l-Glutamine is used as a muscle fuel before it can be converted by the brain to glutamate.

Start with 2 grams (1 level tsp is about 5 grams) twice per day, work up to 5 grams twice per day, or as directed by your healthcare practitioner. L-Glutamine can be mixed in to a smoothie or other liquid.

Again, quit taking it if you develop any symptoms of anxiety or a worsening of existing symptoms. If that happens you should be checked out for sensitivities to MSG L-Glutamine and Aspartic Acid. These are all related compounds and if you are sensitive will require a special diet and avoidance of some supplements. Very few people are sensitive to L-Glutamine, even if sensitive to MSG.

- **<u>Omega 3 Fatty Acids:</u>**

We've all heard that fish oils are good for us, and they are, but they're especially beneficial to gut health. The wrong kind of fats, or too much Omega 6, can actually cause the inflammation we're trying to fix. Omega 3s not only help balance those negative effects, but can help fix the inflammation and the damage it causes.

These are two of the Polyunsaturated Fatty Acids (PUFA), overall we should be cutting back on PUFAs, within that we should be changing the ratio to favor Omega 3s.

Trans fatty acids (trans fats) are not PUFAs, they are an artificial saturated fat; trans fats are especially bad for us and directly cause systemic (throughout the body) inflammation.

Trans fats should be completely avoided by everyone, but especially anyone trying to reduce any sort of inflammation. The good news is that many national restaurant chains are cutting back on their use of trans fats, and it's getting easier to find restaurants that proudly state that they do not cook with trans fats.

To help offset the O3:O6 ratio a little, and help with the inflammation a bad ratio causes, I recommend a good fish oil supplement (such as fermented cod liver oil) as well as a DHA/EPA supplement. If you are working with a doctor you may even ask them about taking 2-3 grams (4-6 capsules) of DHA per day while healing.

A DHA/EPA supplement is certainly a must for anyone trying to fix the lingering inflammation caused by SIBO or SIFO. In order for this to work, you should cut back on Omega 6 fatty acids (vegetable oils, soybean oil, canola oil, etc.) and consume no trans-fat oils (hydrogenated and partially hydrogenated oils).

General Tips for Abdominal Pain

Doctors emphasize the fact that our health, in general, is in great part, dictated by our gut and abdominal health. Abdominal, or gut health, is crucial for your overall well-being because a healthy gut is able to absorb all crucial nutrients you are ingesting with food consumption which aids in less abdominal cramps.

Problems with digestion play a major role in determining your vitality and well-being, also preventing the development of chronic abdominal pains. These top 5 general, perhaps weird, but helpful tips may help you deal with the abdominal pains you may be facing.

Tip #1: Introduce More Fiber to Your Everyday Diet

Talking about the good gut bacteria that protect your intestinal health, you should also note that these bacteria need food just as you do, in order to survive and battle bad bacteria that also reside in your intestines. The "favorite" food of good gut bacteria is actually fiber, which is why it is recommended to introduce more fiber to your diet.

Tip #2: Lower Consumption of Red Meat

Consuming too much red meat may actually harm your health despite the fact that red meat is rich in protein. Of course, you should introduce red meat to your diet, preferably grass-fed and organic, however, try reducing the intake of red meat on the cost of increasing your weekly consumption of recommended fish such as salmon.

Tip #3: Don't Use Antibiotics Unless Necessary
Even if you are forced to use antibiotics due to an infection, your body may be suffering from, and as prescribed by your doctor, it is recommended to avoid using antibiotics unless you really need to. In case you do need antibiotics, it is highly recommended to use probiotics and prebiotics while you are on antibiotic therapy. Antibiotics may destroy the good gut bacteria, lowering the overall population of these bacteria that actually serves the purpose of protecting your health. Prebiotics and probiotics, on the other hand, are set to protect the gut flora of good bacteria.

Tip #4: Allowed Stressful Situations
As weird as it might sound, the number one modern health problem, otherwise known as stress has more effect on your health and your intestinal well-being than you might think. Your body experiences stress as illness or diseases, as previously mentioned, which means that your body immediately becomes a battlefield due to high levels of emotional stress, releasing toxins, and harming your gut health. Allow yourself to take a pause and relax, take a walk, get well rested, and get plenty of sleep.

Tip #5: Drink More Water and Avoid Alcohol
Hydration is the key to a vital body and great health, as, after all, our body is made over 75% of water. Drinking at least 2 liters of water will help you get rid of the toxins that might be piling up in your body, consequently meddling with your gut health and intestinal flora. Avoid alcohol at all costs as alcohol doesn't suit the good bacteria in your gut, even though an occasional glass of red wine is allowed.

Physical Activity and GI Health

Exercise is very important to your long term success in controlling SIBO, yeast infections, and other gastrointestinal dysbiosis. You primarily want to do resistance training, lift heavy things and/or use resistance bands.

This will burn off calories and control blood sugar, both deprive pathogens of the energy they need. As you become more lean (bulking and lean looking muscles for men, mostly long lean looking muscles for women.

This is due to hormonal differences) this lean muscle will continue to burn sugar even when you are at rest. This has a normalizing effect on blood sugar, reducing the chances of pathogens going systemic. Exercise and lean muscle are also known to normalize hormones; balanced hormones help to control pathogens. Try to avoid heavy cardio training, long periods of treadmill, running, etc.

Heavy cardio is very inflammatory and can slow down your healing. It's also not necessary for good health. A good walk at least 3 times per week and a little strength training where possible. You should try to do a little more each week, a slightly longer walk a little more resistance, etc.

Diverticulitis FAQ

1. What is the significance of the Diverticulitis Diet?

While a typical diverticulitis diet, itself, is not considered a sole treatment for diverticulitis, it does strengthen the overall effect of the therapy, and ensures rapid healing and fast improvement in symptoms. In other words, a diverticulitis diet helps people while they are still on the treatment and ensures better healing rates and improvement in symptoms. A diverticulitis diet also eases the burden from the digestive during the diverticulitis treatment.

2. What is a clear fluid diet?

As the name implies, this diet is composed of clear liquids and foods that are liquid at room temperature. These include green tea, fresh fruit juice, clear broth, and gelatin dessert. The clear liquid diet provides the body with salt, liquids, and enough nutrients to function temporarily, **generally for a few days,** until you can eat normal food.

3. What are the side effects or risks involved with a Clear Fluid Diet?

As stated throughout the previous chapters, the clear fluid s does not have a sufficient amount of nutrients, one should not take a clear liquid diet for more than 2-3 days, unless your dietician or the doctor has asked you to do so.

Always remember to consult your nutritionist, doctor, or health care provider for any queries you may have about your clear fluid diet plan.

Your doctor or health care provider will also tell you how much fluid you may have on daily basis.

Important NOTE: a clear fluid diet is not a "well-balanced" diet and is not recommended for otherwise normal individuals

4. <u>When to use the diverticulitis diet?</u>
During "uncomplicated" diverticulosis: An uncomplicated diverticulosis simply means the presence of diverticula in the large intestine (colon), before the stage of inflammation or diverticulitis occurs. Therefore, before the development of "diverticulitis" stage, the recommended diet will be a high fiber diet.

When a patient suffers from severe symptoms, such as lower abdominal pain, fever, vomiting, and constipation, and is considered to be experiencing a flare, the diverticulitis diet is implemented. The recommended diet for this phase is clear liquids and a low-fiber diet to follow (explained in detail in previous chapters).

5. Who gets Diverticulosis and Diverticular infection?
Diverticulosis turns out to be more normal as individual's age, especially in individuals more established than age 50.3 Some individuals with Diverticulosis create diverticulitis, and the quantity of cases is expanding.

In spite of the fact that Diverticular disease is for the most part thought to be a condition found in more seasoned grown-ups, it is turning out to be more regular in individuals more youthful than age 50, the greater part of whom are male.

6. When would a Clear Fluid diet be needed?

A clear fluid diet is indicated in the following conditions:

- When you cannot properly digest (break down) solid foods e.g. dehydration, vomiting, diarrhea, after surgery of intestines, or in certain chronic diseases.
- When experiencing a diverticulitis flare, a clear liquid diet is advised. Symptomatic improvement usually occurs within 2-3 days, at which point patients are recommended to slowly reintroduce fiber to their diet.

7. What is the benefit, if any of a clear fluid diet?

The basic benefit of a clear liquid diet is that it helps one feel better until he or she is able to eat solid food.

8. What is the recommended dose of fiber and water per day?

The recommended intake of fiber is generally:

- Women age 19 to 50 = 25 grams per day
- Women age 50+ = 21 grams per day
- Men age 19 to 50 = 38 grams per day
- Men age 50+ = 30 grams per day

While the recommended water intake is generally:

- Men age 19+ = 12 cups (about 3 liters) per day
- Women age 19+ = 9 cups (about 2 liters) per day

Please contact your doctor to confirm that these values are okay for your specific scenario.

9. Are there any side effects?

Naturally, as a clear liquid diet lacks solid or semi solid food, you may have diarrhea (loose, watery stools), nausea and vomiting (throwing up), and flatulence when you are on this kind of diet.

10. What is fiber?

Fiber is a substance in foods that originates from plants. Fiber diminishes stool so it moves easily through the colon and is less demanding to pass. Solvent fiber disintegrates in water and is found in beans, organic product, and oat items.

Insoluble fiber does not break down in water and is found in entire grain items and vegetables. Both sorts of fiber forestall stoppage. Obstruction is a condition in which a grown-up has less than three solid discharges a week or has defecations with stools that are hard, dry, and little, making them excruciating or hard to pass.

High-fiber foods likewise have numerous advantages in counteracting and controlling incessant maladies, for example, cardiovascular illness, stoutness, diabetes, and disease.

11. What are the symptoms of a Diverticular Infection?

Individuals with diverticulitis may have numerous symptoms, the most widely recognized of which agony in the lower is left half of the stomach area. The torment is normally serious and goes ahead all of a sudden; however, it can likewise be gentle and afterward decline more than a few days. The force of the agony can vacillate.

Diverticulitis may likewise bring about:
- Fevers and chills
- Sickness or heaving
- An adjustment in gut propensities—blockage or the runs
- Diverticular seeping
- As a rule, individuals with Diverticular draining abruptly have a lot of red or maroon-hued blood in their stool.

Diverticular draining may likewise bring about:
- Shortcoming
- Dazedness or discombobulating
- stomach cramping

12. What is a soft diet?
A soft diet, also known as the Low Residue diet, is one that consists of mashed, pureed foods, or foods placed in a sauce for convenient swallowing.

13. When would a soft diet be needed?
Also known as the Low Residue phase of the diet, a soft diet can be used as a short-term step in the progression from liquid to solid foods. In addition, a soft diet is often advised after surgical treatment of diverticulitis. Also, during the transition or recovery phases after a diverticulitis flare, and after any type of jaw, dental, throat, or digestive tract surgery

14. What are the side effects or risks involved with the soft diet?
There are generally no side effects at this stage. However, in some cases, diarrhea has been observed.

What is Diverticular bleeding and Is It Dangerous?

Diverticular bleeding is uncommon. On the off chance that you experience bleeding, it may be serious. Some patients may see their bleeding stop without any form of treatment or seeking medical assistance. Be that as it may, in the event that you notice your rectum bleeding, regardless of the amount, you ought to see a specialist immediately.

A medical professional would be able to discover the site of the bleeding using a colonoscopy in order to stop it from the source. The medical professional may likewise utilize an angiogram or an automated tomography (CT) check to discover the bleeding site.

An angiogram, for those unaware, is a unique sort of x-beam that involves your specialist stringing a dainty, adaptable tube through an extensive corridor, frequently from your crotch to the area that is bleeding.

15. Can Diverticulitis Be Treated or Cured?

A medicinal services supplier may treat the side effects of Diverticulosis with a high fiber eating routine or fiber supplements, prescriptions, and conceivably probiotics. Treatment for Diverticular disease changes, contingent upon whether a man has diverticulitis or other diverticular issues.

With Diverticulitis one would consider:

- **Following a High-fiber diet.** As we have established throughout this guide a high-fiber eating regimen can avert Diverticular illness in individuals who have been diagnosed with diverticulosis. Your healthcare provider may

73

also be able to recommend a moderate increment in dietary fiber to minimize gas and stomach inconvenience.

- **Traditional Medicine.** Various studies recommend the drug mesalazine (Asacol), given either consistently or in cycles, might be successful at decreasing stomach torment and GI manifestations of Diverticulosis. Research has likewise demonstrated that consolidating mesalazine with the anti-infection rifaximin (Xifaxan) can be altogether more powerful than utilizing rifaximin alone to enhance a man's side effects and keep up times of abatement, which means being free of symptoms.
- **Fiber supplements.** Your healthcare provider may also suggest taking a fiber supplement, such as, methylcellulose (Citrucel) or psyllium (Metamucil) one to three times each day. These supplements are accessible as powders, pills, or wafers and give 0.5 to 3.5 grams of fiber for every measurement. Fiber supplements ought to be taken with no less than 8 ounces of water.
- **Probiotics.** Though the effectiveness of proper probiotics is still being researched, probiotics may be useful in treating the symptoms of Diverticulosis. They also prevent the onset of diverticulitis and diminish the possibility of intermittent flares.

What are Probiotics?
Probiotics are live microscopic organisms, similar to those ordinarily found in the GI tract. Probiotics can be found in dietary supplements—in containers, tablets, and

powders—and in a few sustenance, for example, yogurt.

Please Note: To guarantee continued safety and healing, patients are advised to consult with their healthcare professional before embarking on any course of supplements or probiotics.

16. How Can I Tell How Much Fiber is In A Product?

The measure of fiber in a sustenance is recorded on the food nutrition label on the back of the item and can also widely be found in a number of natural products, such as fresh fruits and vegetables.

17. How Much Fiber Do I Need To Add To My General Diet To Be High Fiber?

The general recommended dietary fiber intake in most dietary guides is 14 grams for every 1,000 calories eaten. Following this guide, an average person consuming a 2,000-calorie diet should be consuming 28 grams of fiber daily when on a regular diet.

To figure out the exact number of grams you may be able to push this up to for your specific Diverticulitis diet plan, it is recommended that you consult and work along side a healthcare professional, dietician or nutritionist.

21 Day Action Plan for Diverticulitis

Having a diverticulitis flare can be a stressful and pain filled time. Many times, during your actual flare a clear liquid diet (discussed in more detail below) will help ease your symptoms. Afterwards however, understanding when and how to reintroduce fiber can be tricky as it can the flare to worsen if not done correctly,

Let's explore a 21-day action plan to assist you in reintroducing fiber into your diet safely. Please be sure to consult your doctor on your specific condition before embarking on this action or meal plan.

Phase 1 (Days 1 – 7 of a Flare) – Clear Liquid Diet

While experiencing a diverticulitis flare, or at the first sign of symptoms, it is imperative that you give your digestive tract a break to cleanse and heal itself. During the first few days to a week of your flare or symptoms it is recommended that you consume a Clear Liquid Diet of clear soups, broths, teas and even ice pops.

An example of a recipe you can enjoy during this phase is featured below and you can find many other recipes to mix and match from the recipe section of this cookbook.

Homey Clear Chicken Broth

Yields: 6 cups   Prep: 10 mins.   Cook: 3-1/4 hours
Nutrition per Serving:
245 calories, 14g fat, 8g carbs, 2g fiber, 21g protein

Ingredients:
- Chicken neck (2 lbs)
- celery ribs with leaves (2, cut into chunks)
- carrots (2 medium, cut into chunks)
- onions (2 medium, quartered)
- bay leaves (2)
- rosemary (1/2 teaspoon dried, crushed)
- thyme (1/2 teaspoon dried)
- peppercorns (8 to 10 whole)
- cold water (2 quarts)

Directions:
1. Transfer the bones and vegetables to your stockpot. Top with enough water to cover then allow to slowly come to a boil on high heat.
2. Switch to low heat and simmer for at least 2 hours and up to 12 hours. (The longer it cooks, the more flavor you will get.)
3. Carefully pour the mixture through a fine mesh strainer into a large bowl. Taste and season with salt.
4. Serve hot.

Bone stock with cooked vegetables and a little bit of meat, gives key supplements your body needs, including calcium, magnesium, phosphorus, silicon, sulfur, and that's just the beginning, in an effortlessly processed way.

You may add vegetables to your bone stock including carrots, celery and garlic or for variety; you may include an egg poached in the stock. Furthermore, taste on warm ginger tea a few times every day to lessen aggravation and help in assimilation. Ginger is a healing food that helps your resistant and digestive systems.

For beef, the collagen in the bones separates into gelatin inside around 48 hours, and for chicken it is around 24. You can make soup in less time, yet to get the most out of the bones, I suggest making it in a stewing pot more like 48 hours.

Gelatin has stunning curative properties and even helps people with food sensitivities and hypersensitivities endure these foods all the more effortlessly. It likewise advances probiotic parity, while separating proteins making them less demanding to process. Reality about probiotic and digestive issues is that they make a solid situation in your paunch. During this first period of the diverticulitis diet, devour just clear bone juices, clear crisp squeezes no ash), and calming ginger tea.

Phase 2 (Days 7 – 14 after a Flare) – Low Residue/Fiber Diet

About 7 days after a treated diverticulitis flare, you can proceed onward to phase two of the diverticulitis diet and SLOWLY reintroduce fiber into your diet. We refer to this phase as the Low residue Diet as during this week you will be able to enjoy low fiber meals along with the clear fluids if you so desire.

Juicing new natural foods grown from the ground can give a support of supplements. Vegetables and fruits like watercress, lettuce, apples, grapes, beets and carrots can be used to make juices that can be useful during this stage. Maintain a strategic distance from foods with extreme skins and little seeds as they can aggregate in Diverticular sacs.

One such example recipe of this phase is:

Slow Cooker Salsa Turkey

Yields: 8   Prep: 5 mins.   Cook: 8 hrs.
Nutrition per Serving:
178 calories, 4 g fat, 7 g carbs, 2 g fiber, 27 g protein

Ingredients:
- turkey breasts (2 pounds, boneless and skinless)
- salsa (1 cup)
- tomatoes (1 cup, petite, diced, canned choose low sodium)
- Taco Seasoning (2 tablespoons)
- Celery (1/2 cup, diced fine)
- Carrots (1/2 cup, shredded)
- sour cream (3 tablespoons, reduced fat)

Directions:
1. Add your turkey to your slow cooker. Season your turkey with taco seasoning then top with your salsa and vegetables.
2. Add in ½ cup of water. Set to cook on low 7 hours (internal temperature should be 165°F when done).

3. Shred the turkey with 2 forks, add in sour cream and stir. Enjoy.

Phase 3 (Days 15 – 21 daily life outside of flares) – High Fiber Diet

At the point when your body has adjusted to the foods in the Low Residue Stage, begin to include fiber rich foods including crude products of the soil, and grungy grains, for example, quinoa, dark rice, matured grains, or sprouted lentils.

It is essential to avoid entire nuts and seeds, as they can without much of a stretch get to be caught in the Diverticular, eating additional harm.

While seeds, nuts and popcorn are not the reason for diverticulitis, during this phase in healing, it is best to maintain a strategic distance from them. Once your diverticulitis symptoms have ebbed, you can come back to getting a charge out of these foods, and others, with some restraint.

Listen to your body; if anytime you begin to experience diverticulitis symptoms once more, come back to the past stage. It might take the length of a couple of months to totally recuperate your digestive tract.

An example recipe in this stage is:

Pear Turkey Pita

Yields: 4   Prep: 15 mins.   Cook: 0 mins.
Nutrition per Serving:
221 calories, 3 g fat, 21 g carbs, 2 g fiber, 25 g protein

Ingredients:
- Turkey (2 cups, cooked, cubed)
- Pears (2, medium, unpeeled, chopped)
- Celery (1 stalk, chopped)
- Yogurt (1/3 cup, plain, low fat or non-fat)
- Mayonnaise (1/4 cup, non-fat)
- pita breads (4, round, whole wheat)
- lettuce leaves (4, romaine)

Directions:
1. In a bowl, combine the turkey, celery, and pears. Add mayonnaise and yogurt then combine. Create a pocket by slicing pita.
2. Put the lettuce leaf inside the pita and fill the pocket with 1 cup of mixture in each pita bread.
3. Serve with mixed fruits. Do not include berries).

Maintaining A Balanced Diet Daily To Avoid Flare

As indicated by analysts at the University of Oxford, fiber reduces the danger of Diverticular disease. The study concentrated on fiber from natural products, vegetables, oats, and potatoes. So, over the initial few days of stage four, present high-fiber foods bit by bit, including only one new nourishment each 3-4 days.

As your body adjusts you can start devouring around 25-35 grams of fiber every day, to combat potential flares, while your body heals your digestive tract. Include a few potatoes, sweet potatoes, root vegetables, then gradually attempt some non-prepared grains/beans, for example, oats or lentils.

One important qualification is the contrast between solvent fiber, and insoluble fiber. Dissolvable fiber really holds water and transforms into a gel during the digestive procedure. The gel moderates the processing, considering more prominent assimilation of key supplements. Insoluble fiber, then again, adds mass to stools, permitting foods to all the more rapidly leave your system.

Foods high in dissolvable fiber incorporate oat grain, nuts, seeds, beans, lentils grain, and peas. Insoluble fiber is found in foods including entire grains, wheat grain, and vegetables.

Scientists at the Department of Nutrition at Harvard Medical School found that it is the insoluble fiber that declines hazard for creating Diverticular disease. Be that as it may, don't let this influence you from eating an adjusted diet. You don't need to wipe out dissolvable fiber, nor if you. Keeping up a sound parity of protein, fiber, and crisp leafy foods, is key for keeping diverticulitis from erupting.

Be Sure to Incorporate Supplements That Offer:

Aloe

Aloe, in a juice form, helps in absorption, standardizes pH levels, regularizes bowel handling, and energizes sound digestive microorganisms. It is important to maintain a strategic distance from aloe Vera juice with "aloe latex", as it can cause severe stomach cramping and diarrhea.

12 to 16 ounces for each day of aloe juice is prescribed; any more than that can advance aggravate your system.

Slippery Elm

Local Americans have utilized dangerous elm for quite a long time both remotely, and inside to soothe digestive issues and relieve coughs and sore throats.

Today, it is prescribed to relieve the symptoms of GERD, Crohn's disease, IBS, and digestive miracle. Begin by taking 500 milligrams, 3 times day by day, over the span of the diverticulitis diet. Make sure to take with a full glass of water, or other clear fluid.

Licorice Root

Licorice Root is great for reducing acid levels in your stomach. It can also aid in relieving acid reflux and acting as a mild laxative to clear your colon of waste. This root expands bile, supporting in absorption, while bringing down cholesterol levels. Take 100 milligrams every day while encountering diverticulitis symptoms.

Digestive Enzymes

In addition to healing your colon from diverticulitis, the general objective of the diverticulitis diet, supplements, and way of life changes, is to urge your digestive tract to work ideally.

Digestive enzymes separate foods, making it conceivable to assimilate supplements. People with assimilation issues can take digestive supplements that contain crucial catalysts to encourage absorption.

Probiotics

Live probiotic ought to be added to the diet to invalidate food sensitivities, and ease digestive upset including blockage, gas, and bloating.

Probiotics are sound microscopic organisms that generally line your digestive tract to battle disease. On the off chance that you have diverticulitis you require an influx of these microorganisms to help in the healing of your colon, while preventing disease repeat.

Sample Diverticulitis Meal Plans For Incorporating All Three Stages of The Diet

Let's explore three different sample meal plans using the recipes featured in this book for incorporating everyday meals into the three phases of the diverticulitis diet to successfully recover from and prevent future flares.

There are 52 delicious recipes in the sections that follow so please feel free to mix and match recipes to suit your personal taste and scenarios.

Remember this meal plan is meant to be regarded for informational purposes only. Everybody is different as such their flares and speed of recovery may differ. So be sure to speak to a medical professional to be sure this meal plan would be best for you.

Meal Plan for Phase 1 (Clear Liquids) of the Diverticulitis Meal Plan

This first plan would be very influential to implement during the first seven days of a flare.

Day	Breakfast/ Brunch	Lunch/D inner	Snack	Supper/D essert
Day 1	Cinnamon Orange Tea	Oxtail Bone Broth	Pineapp le Ice Cubes	Frozen Strawberry – Peach Pop
Day 2	Kiwi Cinnamon Tea	Homey Clear Chicken Broth	Iced Tea Ice Cubes	Honey Lemonade Popsicle
Day 3	Cranberry Green Tea	Asian Inspired Wonton Broth	Gala Apple Flavore d Ice Cubes	3- Ingredi ent Sugar Free Gelatin
Day 4	Cinnamon Orange Tea	Oxtail Bone Broth	Pineapp le Ice Cubes	Honey Lemonade Popsicle
Day 5	Kiwi Cinnamon Tea	Homey Clear Chicken Broth	Iced Tea Ice Cubes	3- Ingredi ent Sugar Free Gelatin
Day 6	Cranberry	Asian	Pineapp	Honey

	Green Tea	Inspired Wonton Broth	le Ginger Ice Cubes	Lemonade Popsicle
Day 7	Cinnamon Orange Tea	Asian Inspired Wonton Broth	Gala Apple Flavored Ice Cubes	Frozen Strawberry – Peach Pop

Meal Plans for Phase 2 (Low Residue Meals) of the Diverticulitis Meal Plan

This meal plan would be very influential to implement immediately following the first plan, typically days 7 to 14 following a diverticulitis flare.

Day	Breakfast/ Brunch	Lunch/D inner	Snack	Supper/D essert
Day 8	Pear Pancakes	Pea Tuna Salad	Frozen Strawbe rry – Peach Pop	Vegetable Soup
Day 9	Oatmeal Waffles	Slow Cooker Salsa Turkey	Honey Lemona de Popsicle	Pea Tuna Salad
Day 10	Spinach Frittata	Vegetable Soup	Blackbe rry- Rose Ice Pops	Slow Cooker Salsa Turkey
Day 11	Banana and Pear Pita Pockets	Pea Tuna Salad	Frozen Strawbe rry – Peach Pop	Banana Cocoa Cream
Day 12	Pear Pancakes	Mediterra nean Salmon & Potato salad	Honey Lemona de Popsicle	Oatmeal Cookie Smoothie
Day 13	Oatmeal Waffles	Celery Soup	Blackbe rry- Rose Ice	Peach Smoothie

Day 14	Spinach Frittata	Chicken Cutlets	Pops Frozen Strawberry – Peach Pop	Homemade Pumpkin Pie

Meal Plans for Phase 3 (High Fiber Meals) of the Diverticulitis Meal Plan

This meal plan would be very influential to implement immediately following the second plan, typically days 15 and onwards. It involves reintroducing high fiber meals back int your daily diet and shifting to amore balanced way of eating.

Day	Breakfast/ Brunch	Lunch/D inner	Snack	Supper/D essert
Day 15	Veggie Scramble	Pork & Penne Pasta	Pineapp le Ice Cubes	Almond Salad
Day 16	Overnight Oats	Vegetable Curry	Gala Apple Flavore d Ice Cubes	Nutty Green Salad
Day 17	Pear Turkey Pita	Turkey Florentin e	Iced Tea Ice Cubes	Vegetable Nuttolene Salad
Day 18	Turkey and Avocado Pitas	Bean Enchilada s	Frozen Strawbe rry- Peach Pops	Asian Chicken Salad
Day 19	Veggie Scramble	Black Bean Quesadill as	Pineapp le Ice Cubes	Almond Salad
Day 20	Overnight Oats	Broccoli and Mushroo m Rice	Gala Apple Flavore d Ice	Asian Chicken Salad

Day			Cubes	
Day 21	Pear Turkey Pita	Chicken and Asparagu s Pasta	Iced Tea Ice Cubes	Turkey Florentine

Now that we have explored the general background of diverticulitis to give you a better understanding of the disease, let's dive into our 52 amazingly delicious recipes to get you on your way.

Measurement Conversions

It is important to note that it is virtually impossible to include an all-inclusive conversion table as all foods have slightly different measurements when converted.

KITCHEN CONVERSIONS

LIQUID CONVERSIONS

1/4 TSP	= 1 ML		
1/2 TSP	= 2 ML		
1 TSP	= 5 ML		
3 TSP	= 1 TBL	= 1/2 FL OZ	= 15 ML
2 TBLS	= 1/8 CUP	= 1 FL OZ	= 30 ML
4 TBLS	= 1/4 CUP	= 2 FL OZ	= 60 ML
5 1/3 TBLS	= 1/3 CUP	= 3 FL OZ	= 80 ML
8 TBLS	= 1/2 CUP	= 4 FL OZ	= 120 ML
10 2/3	= 2/3 CUP	= 5 FL OZ	= 160 ML
12 TBLS	= 3/4 CUP	= 6 FL OZ	= 180 ML
16 TBLS	= 1 CUP	= 8 FL OZ	= 240 ML
1 PT	= 2 CUPS	= 16 FL OZ	= 480 ML
1 QT	= 4 CUPS	= 32 FL OZ	= 960 ML
33 FL OZ	= 1000 ML	= 1 L	

Length

METRIC	IMPERIAL
3mm	1/8 inch
6mm	1/4 inch
2.5cm	1 inch
3cm	1 1/4 inch
5cm	2 inches
10cm	4 inches
15cm	6 inches
20cm	8 inches
22.5cm	9 inches
25cm	10 inches
28cm	11 inches

Oven Temperatures

	Fahrenheit	Celsius	Gas Mark
Freezing Water	32°F	0°C	
Room Temp.	68°F	20°C	
Boiling Water	212° F	100°C	
Baking	325° F	160°C	3
	350° F	180°C	4
	375° F	190°C	5
	400° F	200°C	6
	425° F	220°C	7
	450° F	230°C	8
Broiling			Grill

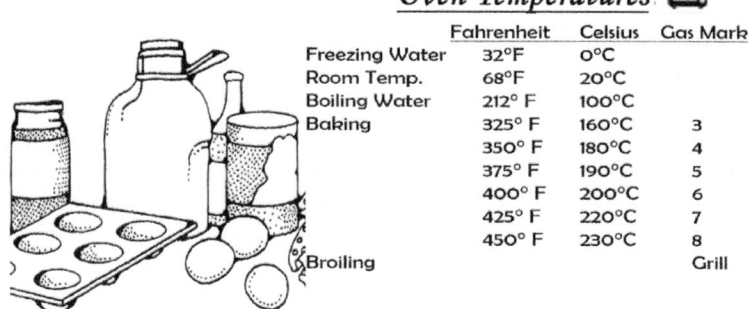

Weight Conversions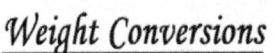

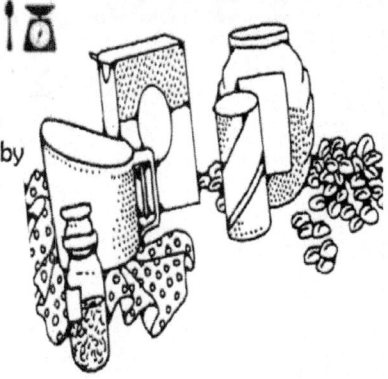

(To convert ounces to grams, multiply the number of ounces by 30.)

1 oz	=	1/16 lb	=	30 g
4 oz	=	1/4 lb	=	120 g
8 oz	=	1/2 lb	=	240 g
12 oz	=	3/4 lb	=	360 g
16 oz	=	1 lb	=	480 g

Conversions for Different Types of Food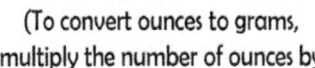

Standard Cup	Fine Powder (like flour)	Grains (like rice)	Granular (like sugar)	Liquid Solids (like butter)	Liquid (eg. milk)
1	140 g	150 g	190 g	200 g	240 ml
3/4	105 g	113 g	143 g	150 g	180 ml
2/3	93 g	100 g	125 g	133 g	160 ml
1/2	70 g	75 g	95 g	100 g	120 ml
1/3	47 g	50 g	63 g	67 g	80 ml
1/4	35 g	38 g	48 g	50 g	60 ml
1/8	18 g	19 g	24 g	25 g	30 ml

PHASE 1 RECIPES:
Clear Fluids

Clear Broths & Stocks

1. *Homey Clear Chicken Broth*

Yields: 6 cups   Prep: 10 mins.   Cook: 3-1/4 hours

Nutrition per Serving:

245 calories, 14g fat, 8g carbs, 2g fiber, 21g protein

Ingredients:
- Chicken neck (2 lbs)
- celery ribs with leaves (2, cut into chunks)
- carrots (2 medium, cut into chunks)
- onions (2 medium, quartered)
- bay leaves (2)
- rosemary (1/2 teaspoon dried, crushed)
- thyme (1/2 teaspoon dried)
- peppercorns (8 to 10 whole)
- cold water (2 quarts)

Directions:
1. Transfer the bones and vegetables to your stockpot. Top with enough water to cover then allow to slowly come to a boil on high heat.
2. Switch to low heat and simmer for at least 2 hours and up to 12 hours. (The longer it cooks, the more flavor you will get.)
3. Carefully pour the mixture through a fine mesh strainer into a large bowl. Taste and season with salt.
4. Serve hot.

2. *Oxtail Bone Broth*

Yields: 8 cups   Prep: 15 mins.   Cook: 12 hours

Nutrition per Serving:

576 calories, 48 g fat, 8 g carbs, 0 g fiber, 24 g protein

Ingredients:

- Oxtail (2 Pounds)
- Onion (1, chopped in quarters)
- celery stalks (2, chopped in half)
- carrots (2, chopped in half)
- garlic cloves (3, whole)
- bay leaves (2)
- apple cider vinegar (2 Tablespoons)
- salt (1 Tablespoon)
- peppercorns (1/2 Tablespoon)
- filtered water (enough to cover bones)

Directions:

1. Transfer the bones and vegetables to your stockpot. Top with enough water to cover then allow to slowly come to a boil on high heat.
2. Switch to low heat and simmer for at least 2 hours and up to 12 hours. (The longer it cooks, the more flavor you will get.)
3. Carefully pour the mixture through a fine mesh strainer into a large bowl. Taste and season with salt.
4. Serve hot.

3. *Asian Inspired Wonton Broth*

Yields: 1-gallon   Prep: 5 mins. Cook: 1 hour 35 mins.

Nutrition per Serving:
181 calories, 7 g fat, 14 g carbs, 1 g fiber, 14g protein

Ingredients:
- chicken thigh (1, skin on)
- carrot (1, coarsely chopped)
- celery (1 stalk, coarsely chopped)
- onion (1 small, quartered)
- ginger (3 dime-sized pieces)
- Kosher salt (2 tablespoons)
- Turmeric (1/4 teaspoon)
- MSG, (1/8 teaspoon, don't leave it out)
- Peppercorns (5 white, black can be substituted)
- Water (1 gallon)

Directions:
1. Transfer all your ingredients to your stockpot. Top with enough water to cover then allow to slowly come to a boil on high heat.
2. Switch to low heat and simmer for at least 1 hours and 30 minutes.
3. Carefully pour the mixture through a fine mesh strainer into a large bowl.
4. Taste and season with salt. Serve hot.

Pulpless Fruit & Vegetable Juices

4. Homemade No Pulp Orange Juice

Yields: 1 ½ cups   Prep: 5 mins. Cook: 0 mins.
Nutrition per Serving:
50 calories, 0.2 g fat, 11.5 g carbs, g fiber, 0.8 g protein

Ingredients:
- Oranges (4)

Directions:
1. Lightly squeeze the oranges on a hard surface to soften the exterior. Slice each in half.
2. Squeeze each orange over a fine mesh strainer.
3. Gently press the pulp to extract all possible liquid.
4. Serve over ice. Enjoy!

5. _Apple Orange Juice_

Yields: 2   Prep: 5 mins. Cook: 0 mins.
Nutrition per Serving:
180 calories, 1 g fat, 43 g carbs, 1 g fiber, 2 g protein

Ingredients:
- Apple (1 Gala, peeled, cored, sliced)
- Oranges (2, peeled, halved, seeded)
- Honey (2 tsp, optional)
- Water (3/4 cup)

Directions:
1. Squeeze each orange over a fine mesh strainer.
2. Gently press the pulp to extract as much liquid as possible.
3. Add in your apple, water, and orange juice in your blender and blend.
4. Set a fine mesh strainer a bowl. Before transferring your juice into the strainer.
5. Once again, gently press the pulp to remove all possible liquid then discard pulp.
6. Stir in your honey then serve over ice.

6. *Pineapple Mint Juice*

Yields: 4   Prep: 5 mins. Cook: 0 mins.
Nutrition per Serving:
78 calories, 1 g fat, 22 g carbs, 2 g fiber, 1 g protein

Ingredients:
- pineapple (3 cups, cored and sliced, chunks)
- mint leaves (10 to 12, or to taste)
- sugar, or to taste (2 tablespoons, optional)
- water (1 1/2 cups)
- ice cubes (1 cup)

Directions:
1. Add all your ingredients into your blender, and blend.
2. Set a fine mesh strainer a bowl. Before transferring your juice into the strainer.
3. Gently press the pulp to extract all possible liquid then discard pulp.
4. Serve over ice. Enjoy!

7. *Pineapple Ice Cubes*

Yields: 24 ice cubes Prep: 4 hrs. 10 mins.   Cook: 0 mins.

Nutrition per Serving:
70 calories, 0 g fat, 18 g carbs, 2 g fiber, 1 g protein

Ingredients:

- Pineapple Juice (3 cups, unsweetened).

Directions:
1. Fill your empty ice trays with your juice.
2. Set to freeze for at least 3 hours until frozen.
3. Transfer your flavored ice cubes to freezer bags.
4. Keep them in the freezer until ready to serve.

8. Gala Apple Flavored Ice Cubes

Yields: 24 ice cubes Prep: 4 hrs. 10 mins.   Cook: 0 mins.

Nutrition per Serving:
83 calories,1 g fat, 21 g carbs, 2 g fiber, 1 g protein

Ingredients:

- Apple (2, Gala)
- Honey (4 tsp.)
- Water (3 cups)

Directions:
1. Add all your ingredients into your blender, and blend.
2. Set a fine mesh strainer a bowl. Before transferring your juice into the strainer.
3. Gently press the pulp to extract all possible liquid then discard pulp.
4. Fill your empty ice trays with your juice.
5. Set to freeze for at least 3 hours until frozen.
6. Transfer your flavored ice cubes to freezer bags.
7. Keep them in the freezer until ready to serve.

9. _Iced Tea Ice Cubes_

Yields: 24 ice cubes Prep: 4 hrs. 10 mins.   Cook: 0 mins.

Nutrition per Serving:
20 calories, 0 g fat, 3 g carbs, 0 g fiber, 0 g protein

Ingredients:

- Iced Tea (3 cups, unsweetened)

Directions:

1. Fill your empty ice trays with your juice.
2. Set to freeze for at least 3 hours until frozen.
3. Transfer your flavored ice cubes to freezer bags.
4. Keep them in the freezer until ready to serve.

10. Blackberry-Rose Ice Pops

Yields: 10   Prep: 25 mins.   Cook: 5 hrs.
Nutrition per Serving:
112 calories, 0 g fat, 30g carbs, 5 g fiber, 1 g protein

Ingredients:
- cane sugar (9 tbsp., organic)
- Water (9 tbsp., for simple syrup)
- blackberries (6 1/2 cups)
- lemon juice (1 tbsp.)
- rosewater (1 tsp.)
- Water (1 cup)

Directions:
1. Create a simple syrup by heating sugar and the water for the simple syrup over medium heat.
2. Allow the mixture to simmer, stirring until the sugar dissolves. Set to cool (about 10 minutes).
3. Add all your ingredients into your blender, and blend.
4. Set a fine mesh strainer a bowl. Before transferring your juice into the strainer.
5. Gently press the pulp to extract all possible liquid then discard pulp.
6. Pour your juice into your ice-pop molds, filling each three quarters of the way.
7. Add in your ice pop sticks then set to freeze for at least 5 hours or until solid. Unmold and enjoy.

11. *Frozen Strawberry-Peach Pops*

Yields: 5   Prep: 5 mins. Cook: 0 mins.
Nutrition per Serving:
102 calories, 1 g fat, 12g carbs, 2 g fiber,2 g protein

Ingredients:
- Sugar (1/2 cup)
- Strawberries (6 oz.)
- Peaches (6 oz.)
- Water (4 oz.)
- Lemon Juice (1 tbsp.)

Directions:
1. Create a simple syrup by heating sugar and water over medium heat.
2. Allow the mixture to simmer, stirring until the sugar dissolves. Set to cool (about 10 minutes).
3. Add all your ingredients into your blender, and blend.
4. Set a fine mesh strainer a bowl. Before transferring your juice into the strainer.
5. Gently press the pulp to extract all possible liquid then discard pulp.
6. Pour your juice into your ice-pop molds, filling each three quarters of the way.
7. Add in your ice pop sticks then set to freeze for at least 5 hours or until solid. Unmold and enjoy.

12. Honey Lemonade Popsicles

Yields: 8   Prep: 5 mins. Cook: 0 mins.
Nutrition per Serving:
36 calories, 3 g fat, 3 g carbs, 1g fiber, 3 g protein

Ingredients:
- Honey (1/2 cup)
- Lemon Juice (12 oz.)
- Water (6 oz.)

Directions:
1. Create honey water by heating honey and over medium heat.
2. Allow the mixture to simmer, stirring until the honey melts. Set to cool (about 10 minutes).
3. In a spouted container, combine all your ingredients.
4. Pour your juice into your ice-pop molds, filling each three quarters of the way.
5. Add in your ice pop sticks then set to freeze for at least 5 hours or until solid. Unmold and enjoy.

Gelatin

13. *3-Ingredient Sugar Free Gelatin*

Yields:6-8   Prep: 5 mins. Cook: 4hrs.
Nutrition per Serving:
17 calories, 0 g fat, 4 g carbs, 0 g fiber, 0 g protein

Ingredients:

- Water (1/4 cup, room temperature)
- Water (1/4 cup, hot)
- Gelatin (1 tbsp.)
- Orange Juice (1 cup, unsweetened)

Directions:

1. Combine your gelatin and room temperature water, stirring until fully dissolved.
2. Stir in your hot water then leave to rest for about 2 minutes.
3. Add in your juice and stir until combined.
4. Transfer to serving size containers then place on a tray in the refrigerator to set for about 4 hours.
5. Enjoy!

14. Cran - Kombucha Jell-O

Yields: 6   Prep: 5 mins. Cook: 4hrs.

Nutrition per Serving:
13 calories, 0 g fat, 1 g carbs, 0 g fiber, 0 g protein

Ingredients:

- Water (1/4 cup, room temperature)
- Hot Water (1/4 cup)
- Gelatin (1 tbsp.)
- Cranberry kombucha (1 cup, unsweetened)

Directions:

1. Combine your gelatin and room temperature water, stirring until fully dissolved.
2. Stir in your hot water then leave to rest for about 2 minutes.
3. Add in your kombucha and stir until combined.
4. Transfer to serving size containers then place on a tray in the refrigerator to set for about 4 hours.
5. Enjoy!

15. *Strawberry Gummies*

Yields: 20-40 mini gummies   Prep: 5 mins.
Cook: 4 hrs.
Nutrition per Serving:
3 calories, 0 g fat, 0 g carbs, 0 g fiber, 0 g protein

Ingredients:
- Strawberries (1 cup, hulled, chopped)
- Water (3/4 cup)
- Gelatin (2 tbsp.)

Directions:
1. Set your water and berries on to boil on high heat. /remove from heat as soon as the mixture begins to boil.
2. Transfer to your blender and blend. Add in your gelatin then blend once more.
3. Pour your mixture into a silicone gummy mold.
4. Place on a tray in the refrigerator to set for about 4 hours.
5. Enjoy!

Flavored Tea

16. Kiwi Cinnamon Tea

Yields: 4   Prep: 5 mins. Cook: 25 mins.
Nutrition per Serving:
101 calories, 1 g fat, 27 g carbs, 1 g fiber, 1 g protein

Ingredients:
- Kiwi (1 cup, chopped)
- cinnamon sticks (3)
- water (1-quart)
- Earl Grey tea (2 bags)
- Honey (⅓ cup)

Directions:
1. In a large saucepan over high heat, add in the Kiwi, cinnamon sticks, and water then boil.
2. Switch to medium heat and simmer for 15 minutes. Switch off the heat and add the tea bags. Steep for 10 minutes.
3. Using a slotted spoon, remove the solid ingredients. Add the honey and stir well. Add more honey, if desired.
4. Serve hot. If there are any leftovers, store in an airtight container in the refrigerator for up to 5 days. Can be served cold or reheat in the microwave for 1 minute until hot.

17. *Cranberry Green Tea*

Yields: 4   Prep: 5 mins. Cook: 25 mins.
Nutrition per Serving:
95 calories, 0 g fat, 26 g carbs, 1 g fiber, 1 g protein

Ingredients:
- Cranberry (½ cup)
- water (1-quart)
- green tea (2 bags)
- honey (⅓ cup)

Directions:
1. In a large saucepan over high heat, add in the cranberries, and water then boil.
2. Switch to medium heat and simmer for 15 minutes. Switch off the heat and add the tea bags. Steep for 10 minutes.
3. Using a slotted spoon, remove the solid ingredients. Add the honey and stir well. Add more honey, if desired.
4. Serve hot. If there are any leftovers, store in an airtight container in the refrigerator for up to 5 days. Can be served cold or reheat in the microwave for 1 minute until hot.

18. Cinnamon Orange Tea

Yields: 4   Prep: 5 mins. Cook: 25 mins.
Nutrition per Serving:
101 calories, 1 g fat, 27 g carbs, 1 g fiber, 1 g protein

Ingredients:
- orange (1 cup, wedges)
- cinnamon (3 sticks)
- water (1-quart)
- Earl Grey tea (2 bags)
- Honey (⅓ cup)

Directions:
1. In a large saucepan over high heat, add in the orange, cinnamon sticks, and water then boil.
2. Switch to medium heat and simmer for 15 minutes.
3. Switch off the heat and add the tea bags. Steep for 10 minutes.
4. Using a slotted spoon, remove the solid ingredients. Add the honey and stir well. Add more honey, if desired.
5. Serve hot. If there are any leftovers, store in an airtight container in the refrigerator for up to 5 days. Can be served cold or reheat in the microwave for 1 minute until hot.

PHASE 2 RECIPES: Low Residue Meals

19. _Oatmeal Waffles_

Yields: 2-3   Prep: 10 mins.   Cook: 15 mins.
Nutrition per Serving:
404 calories, 7 g fat, 47 g carbs, 6 g fiber, 15 g protein

Ingredients:
- Quick Oats (1 1/2 cups)
- White flour (1/2 cup, refined)
- baking powder (1 tbs)
- cinnamon (1 tbs)
- nutmeg (1 tsp)
- egg (1)
- banana (1, mashed)
- honey (1 tbs)
- milk (1 1/2 cups)
- cooking spray (Non-stick)

Directions:
1. In a large bowl mix together oatmeal, cinnamon, baking powder, whole wheat flour, and nutmeg. Set aside.
2. In a separate bowl, mix egg, banana, honey, and milk. Mix dry mixture into wet mixture. Preheat waffle iron.
3. Spray with non-stick cooking spray.
4. Pour less than 1/4 cup batter into hot pan for each waffle.
5. Cook until puffy and dry around edges. Turn and cook other side until golden.

20. *Spinach Frittata*

Yields: 4   Prep: 10 mins.   Cook: 30 mins.
Nutrition per Serving:
106 calories, 8 g fat, 7 g carbs, 2 g fiber, 3 g protein

Ingredients:
- olive oil (2 tsp)
- red pepper (1 cup, seeded, chopped)
- garlic (1 clove, minced)
- spinach leaves (3 cups, chopped)
- eggs (4, large, beaten)
- salt (1/2 tsp)
- Parmesan cheese (1/4 cup, freshly grated)

Directions:
1. Preheat oven to 350 degrees. In a non-stick oven pan, heat 1 tsp olive oil over medium heat.
2. Cook red peppers and garlic until vegetables are soft (about 10 minutes). In medium bowl, combine eggs and spinach and salt; set aside.
3. Add remaining 1 tsp olive oil into pan with vegetables and add in the egg mixture.
4. Turn the heat to medium and cook for 15 mins. Sprinkle Parmesan cheese over top of mixture and broil for an additional 4 minutes.

21. Banana and Pear Pita Pockets

Yields: 1   Prep: 5 mins. Cook: 25 mins.
Nutrition per Serving:
402 calories, 2 g fat, 87 g carbs, 11 g fiber, 14 g protein

Ingredients:
- Banana (1/2 small, peeled, sliced)
- pita bread (1, round, made with refined white flour)
- pear (1/2, small, peeled, seedless, cored, cooked, sliced)
- cottage cheese (1/4 cup, low fat

Directions:
1. Combine banana, pear, and cottage cheese in a small bowl. Slice pita to make a pocket. Fill pita pocket with mixture. Serve.

22. Pear Pancakes

Yields: 4   Prep: 5 mins. Cook: 15 mins.
Nutrition per Serving:
174 calories, 2 g fat, 34 g carbs, 2 g fiber, 5 g protein

Ingredients:
- Eggs (2)
- Pear (1 cup, peeled mashed)
- Cinnamon (1 tsp)
- Sugar (2 tsp)
- Refined white flour (1 1/2 cup)
- flour (1/2 cup, whole-wheat)
- baking powder (2 tsp)
- vanilla (2 tsp)
- cooking spray (Non-stick)

Directions:
1. In a medium bowl, beat eggs until fluffy. Add baking powder, cinnamon, vanilla, sugar, flours, and pear, and continue to stir just until smooth.
2. Heat griddle or non-stick pan over medium heat.
3. Spray with non-stick cooking spray. Pour a sizeable amount of batter that you want your pancake to be into the hot pan.
4. Cook pancakes until puffy and dry around edges.
5. Turn and cook other side until golden. Serve pancakes with additional pear if desired.

23. Mediterranean Salmon and Potato Salad

Yields: 4   Prep: 15 mins.   Cook: 18 mins.
Nutrition per Serving:
463 calories, 4 g fat, 75 g carbs, 18 g fiber, 34g protein

Ingredients:

- red potatoes (1 lb., peeled, cut into wedges)
- extra virgin olive oil (1/2 cup, plus 2 tbs more)
- balsamic vinegar (2 tbs)
- fresh rosemary (1 tbs, minced)
- peas (2 cups, cooked, drained)
- salmon fillets (4, 4 oz each)
- lemon juice (2 tbs)
- salt (1/4 tsp)
- English cucumbers (2 cups, sliced, seedless)

Directions:

1. In a medium saucepan, bring water to a boil and cook potatoes until tender, about 10 minutes.
2. Drain and pour potatoes back into pan. To make dressing, in a small bowl, whisk together 1/2 cup of olive oil, vinegar and rosemary.

3. Combine potatoes and peas with dressing. Set aside. In a separate medium pan, heat the remaining 2 tbs of olive oil over medium heat.
4. Add salmon fillets and sprinkle with lemon juice and salt.
5. Cook for 4 minutes on both side or until fish flakes easily. To serve, place cucumber slices on a serving platter top with potato salad and fish fillets.

24. Celery Soup

Yields: 4   Prep: 8 mins. Cook: 10 mins.
Nutrition per Serving:
51 calories, 3 g fat, 4 g carbs, 2 g fiber, 2 g protein

Ingredients:

- olive oil (1 tbs)
- garlic cloves (3, minced)
- celery (2 lbs., fresh, chopped into
- one-inch pieces.)
- vegetable stock (6 cups)
- salt (1 tsp)

Directions:

1. Reserve celery tops for later use. Heat up the oil over medium heat in a soup pot.
2. Cook garlic until softened, about 3-5 minutes. Add celery stalks, salt and vegetable stock and bring to a boil.
3. Cover and reduce heat to low and simmer until celery softens. Let the soup cool for a bit then and puree with a hand blender.
4. Add and cook the celery tops on medium heat for 5 minutes.

25. *Pea Tuna Salad*

Yields: 4   Prep: 1 hr. 15 mins. Cook: 10 mins.
Nutrition per Serving:
246 calories, 13 g fat, 11 g carbs, 1 g fiber, 22 g protein

Ingredients:

- Peas (3 lbs., cooked)
- mayonnaise (1/2 cup, low fat)
- tarragon vinegar (1/3 cup)
- honey Dijon mustard (1 tsp)
- shallots (2 small, sliced thinly)
- tuna fish (2 (6 oz) cans, drained)
- sprigs fresh tarragon (2 small, chopped finely)

Directions:

1. In a large bowl, combine mayonnaise, vinegar and mustard. Add tuna fish, shallots and peas; toss to coat with dressing.
2. Cover and refrigerate one hour prior to serving. Garnish with fresh tarragon and serve.

26. Vegetable Soup

Yields: 4   Prep: 15 mins.   Cook: 1 hr. 5 mins.
Nutrition per Serving:
242 calories, 8 g fat, 34 g carbs, 13 g fiber, 12 g protein

Ingredients:

- extra virgin olive oil (2 tbsp)
- garlic cloves (4, chopped finely)
- celery stalks (2, sliced finely)
- carrots (2, sliced finely)
- water (6 cups or chicken broth)
- thyme (1/4 tsp)
- rosemary (1/4 tsp)
- bay leaf (1)
- Peas (1 can (14 oz)
- salt (1/2 tsp)

Directions:

1. Heat up the oil over medium heat in a soup pot. Add garlic, celery, and carrots and continue to cook for 5 minutes, stirring occasionally.
2. Add water or chicken broth, thyme, rosemary and bay leaf and cook until it comes to a boil.
3. Reduce heat and cover and simmer gently for about 45-60 minutes. Add peas and season with salt.
4. Let soup cool slightly, remove bay leaf and puree with a hand blender, until creamy. Serve in warmed soup bowls.

27. *Italian Styled Stuffed Zucchini Boats*

Yields: 6   Prep: 5 mins. Cook: 25 mins.
Nutrition per Serving:
298 calories, 17 g fat, 14 g carbs, 2 g fiber, 25 g protein

Ingredients:

- zucchini (6 large)
- olive oil
- kosher salt
- freshly ground black pepper
- garlic powder (1/4 tsp.)
- yellow onion (1 small, diced)
- garlic (2 cloves, minced)
- ground turkey (1 lb.)
- crush tomatoes (1 (28 oz.) can)
- mozzarella cheese (4 oz., shredded)
- parmesan cheese (1 oz., freshly grated)
- flat leaf parsley for garnish

Directions:

1. Turn your oven on and allow to preheat up to 425 degrees F and lightly grease a 9x13-inch baking dish with cooking spray.
2. Slice the zucchini in half lengthwise and then scoop out the seeds. Brush with olive oil and season with salt, pepper and garlic powder.
3. Roast in the prepared dish for 20 minutes, or until it begins to soften.
4. Meanwhile, sauté the onions and garlic in a ½ tbsp of olive oil over medium high heat in a large skillet.
5. Cook for 3-4 minutes, then add the ground turkey and brown. Add the tomatoes and bring to a boil.
6. Reduce heat to medium and then let simmer until the zucchini are done. Stir in ½ tsp salt and pepper to taste.
7. Fill the zucchini boats with the meat mixture and sprinkle on shredded cheese.
8. Set to bake for about 5 minutes or at least until the cheese you added has melted, about 3-5 minutes.
9. Serve hot, garnished with parmesan cheese and parsley.

☐

28. Chicken Cutlets

Yields: 4   Prep: 15 mins.   Cook: 15 mins.
Nutrition per Serving:
549 calories, 6 g fat, 7g carbs, 1 g fiber, 114g protein

Ingredients:
- red wine vinegar (4 tsp)
- minced garlic (2 tsp)
- dried sage leaves (2 tsp)
- chicken breast cutlets (1 pound)
- Salt and pepper, to taste
- flour (1/4 cup, refined white)
- olive oil (2 tsp)
- reduced-sodium fat-free chicken broth (1/2 cup)
- lemon juice (1 tbs)

Directions:
1. Lay a good amount of plastic wrap on the kitchen counter; sprinkle with half the combine sage, garlic and vinegar.
2. Put the chicken breast on the plastic wrap; sprinkle with the rest of the vinegar mixture. Season lightly with pepper and salt.
3. Cover the chicken with a second sheet of plastic wrap. Use a kitchen mallet to pound the breast until it is flattened. Let stand 5 minutes.
4. Coat the chicken on both sides with flour. In a skillet, heat up the oil over medium heat.
5. Add half of the chicken breast and cook for 1 ½ minutes or until it is browned on bottom.
6. Turn on the other side and let it cook for 3 minutes.

7. Remove the chicken breast and place it on a to oven-proof serving platter so that you can keep warm.
8. Do the same step with the rest of the cutlets. Heat up the lemon juice and the broth to a boil in skillet.
9. Reduce the liquid by half. Pour mixture over the chicken breast; serve immediately.

29. Slow Cooker Salsa Turkey

Yields: 8   Prep: 5 mins. Cook: 8 hrs.
Nutrition per Serving:
178 calories, 4 g fat, 7 g carbs, 2 g fiber, 27 g protein

Ingredients:
- turkey breasts (2 pounds, boneless and skinless)
- salsa (1 cup)
- tomatoes (1 cup, petite, diced, canned choose low sodium)
- Taco Seasoning (2 tablespoons)
- Celery (1/2 cup, diced fine)
- Carrots (1/2 cup, shredded)
- sour cream (3 tablespoons, reduced fat)

Directions:
1. Add your turkey to your slow cooker. Season your turkey with taco seasoning then top with your salsa and vegetables.
2. Add in ½ cup of water. Set to cook on low 7 hours (internal temperature should be 165°F when done).
3. Shred the turkey with 2 forks, add in sour cream and stir. Enjoy.

☐

30. Sriracha Lime Chicken & Apple Salad

Yields: 4   Prep: 10 mins.   Cook: 15 mins.
Nutrition per Serving:
484 calories, 28 g fat, 32g carbs, 8 g fiber, 30 g protein

Ingredients:
Sriracha Lime Chicken:

- chicken breasts (2 organic)
- sriracha (3 tbsp.)
- lime (1, juiced)
- fine sea salt (1/4 tsp.)
- freshly ground pepper (1/4 tsp.)

Fruit Salad:

- apple (4, peeled, cored, diced)
- grape tomatoes (1 cup organic)
- red onion (1/3 cup, finely chopped)

Lime Vinaigrette:

- light olive oil (1/3 cup)
- apple cider vinegar (1/4 cup)
- limes (2, juiced)
- dash fine sea salt

Directions:

1. Use your salt and pepper to season the chicken on both sides. Spread on the sriracha and lime and let the chicken sit for 20 minutes.
2. Cook the chicken for 3-4 minutes per side over medium heat, or until done. Grill the apple with the chicken.
3. Meanwhile, whisk together the dressing and season to taste. Dress the salad and serve as a side to the chicken and apple.

Low Residue Smoothie & Dessert

31. Banana Cocoa Cream

Yields: 4   Prep: 4 hrs.   Cook: 0 mins.
Nutrition per Serving:
0.1 calories, 1 g fat, 7 g carbs, 1g fiber, 0 g protein

Ingredients:
- Banana (1, mashed)
- cocoa powder, to taste
- stevia, to taste (optional)

Directions:
1. Mix one mashed banana with stevia and cocoa powder. You may blend these together or use a food processor for best results.
2. Freeze in a sealed container for 2-4 hours.

32. *Honey Banana Smoothie*

Yields: 1   Prep: 15 mins.   Cook: 0 mins.
Nutrition per Serving:
471 calories, 8 g fat, 75 g carbs, 4 g fiber, 23g protein

Ingredients:
- Banana (1, medium)
- Milk (1 cup, low fat)
- Yogurt (1/2 cup, nonfat, plain)
- Refined cereal (1/4 cup)
- vanilla extract (1 tsp)
- honey (2 tsp)
- ice (1/2 cup)
- cinnamon (1 dash)

Directions:
1. In a blender put all ingredients and process until smooth. Garnish with cinnamon.

33. Oatmeal Cookie Smoothie

Yields: 1   Prep: 5 mins. Cook: 0 mins.

Nutrition per Serving:

336 calories, 11 g fat, 54 g carbs, 5 g fiber, 10 g protein

Ingredients:

- yellow banana (1 sliced and frozen)
- milk (¾ cup)
- ice (¼ cup)
- rolled oats (2 tbsp.)
- almond butter (2 tsp.)
- vanilla (1/8 tsp.)
- cinnamon (½ tsp.)
- Small sprinkle ground nutmeg optional

Directions:

1. Add all your ingredients to your blender then allow to process until you achieve a smooth consistency.

34. *Peach Smoothie*

Yields: 1   Prep: 10 mins.   Cook: 0 mins.
Nutrition per Serving:
367 calories, 8 g fat, 44 g carbs, 2 g fiber, 23 g protein

Ingredients:

- Peaches (1/2 cup, peeled, cooked)
- milk (1 cup, non-fat)
- yogurt (1/2 cup, non-fat, peach flavoured)
- flakes (1/4 cup, refined cereal)
- vanilla extract (1 tsp)
- honey (1 tsp, optional)
- ice (1/2 cup)

Directions:

1. In a blender put all ingredients and process until smooth and creamy.

35. Homemade Pumpkin Pie

Yields: 10   Prep: 5 mins. Cook: 45 mins.
Nutrition per Serving:
342 calories, 1 g fat, 42 g carbs, 1 g fiber, 5 g protein

Ingredients:
Crust:

- 1 Pie crust (All butter, 9-inch, chilled)

Filling:

- pumpkin purée (1, 15- ounce, can)
- sugar (¾ cup)
- eggs (2 large, at room temperature)
- lactose-free evaporated milk (11- ounces)
- cinnamon (1 teaspoon)
- ginger (½ teaspoon, ground)
- salt (1/4 teaspoon)
- cloves (¼ teaspoon, ground)

Directions:

1. Position your rack in the center of oven. Set to preheat to 425F. Whisk together your sugar, eggs, and pumpkin.
2. Whisk in your salt, cinnamon, ginger, clove and evaporated milk until smooth.
3. Add filling to your crust and set to bake (about 15 minutes). Switch the oven temperature to 350F and allow to bake at the lower temperature until set (about 45 minutes).

4. Cool completely then serve.

PHASE 3 RECIPES: High Fiber Meals

36. _Pear Turkey Pita_

Yields: 4   Prep: 15 mins.   Cook: 0 mins.

Nutrition per Serving:

221 calories, 3 g fat, 21 g carbs, 2 g fiber, 25 g protein

Ingredients:

- Turkey (2 cups, cooked, cubed)
- Pears (2, medium, unpeeled, chopped)
- Celery (1 stalk, chopped)
- Yogurt (1/3 cup, plain, low fat or non-fat)
- Mayonnaise (1/4 cup, non-fat)
- pita breads (4, round, whole wheat)
- lettuce leaves (4, romaine)

Directions:

1. In a bowl, combine the turkey, celery, and pears. Add mayonnaise and yogurt then combine. Create a pocket by slicing pita.
2. Put the lettuce leaf inside the pita and fill the pocket with 1 cup of mixture in each pita bread.
3. Serve with mixed fruits. Do not include berries).

37. *Overnight Oats*

Yields: 4   Prep: 5 mins. Cook: 0 mins.
Nutrition per Serving:
267 calories, 16 g fat, 34 g carbs, 4 g fiber, 4g protein

Ingredients:
- Almond Milk (1 cup)
- Fruit of choice (1/2 cup)
- Gluten-free Oats (1 cup)
- ½ tbsp Honey

Directions:
1. Mix 1 cup oats with 2/3 cup almond milk. Add fruit and honey.
2. Leave in refrigerator overnight in a mason jar or similar sealable container. Mix well in the morning before eating.

38. *Veggie Scramble*

Yields: 1   Prep: 5 mins. Cook: 0 mins.
Nutrition per Serving:
157 calories, 6 g fat, 15 g carbs, 6 g fiber, 16 g protein

Ingredients:
- Eggs (2)
- Spinach (1 cup)
- Tomato (1 medium)
- Spices of your choice (to taste)
- Cooking spray

Directions:
1. Mix eggs, spinach, and chopped tomato in a bowl.
2. Spray a pan with cooking spray and pour bowl contents onto pan when hot. Cook until eggs are no longer runny.

39. *Turkey and Avocado Pitas*

Yields: 4   Prep: 10 mins.   Cook: 0 mins.

Nutrition per Serving:

277 calories, 11 g fat, 10 g carbs, 4 g fiber, 30 g protein

Ingredients:

- Turkey (2 cups, cooked, cubed)
- avocado (1 medium, chopped)
- red beans (1 (14 oz.) can, drained and rinsed)
- lemon juice (1 tsp)
- tomatoes (1 cup, seeded, chopped)
- low fat cottage cheese (1 cup)
- whole wheat pita bread (4 round)

Directions:

1. In a large mixing bowl, combine turkey, avocado, red beans, lemon juice, tomatoes, and cottage cheese.
2. Slice the pita bread to make a pocket and spoon in the turkey mixture. Serve.

High Fiber Vegetarian Meals

40. Bean Enchiladas

Yields: 4   Prep: 15 mins.   Cook: 20 mins.
Nutrition per Serving:
231 calories, 2 g fat, 51 g carbs, 13 g fiber, 12 g protein

Ingredients:
- Red beans, (1, 14 oz can, drained rinsed and mashed)
- low- fat cheddar cheese, (2 cups, shredded)
- onion (1/2 cup, chopped)
- black olives, (1/4 cup)
- tomato sauce (2 cups)
- garlic salt (2 tsp)
- whole wheat tortillas (8 medium)

Directions:
1. Preheat oven to 350F degrees. In a bowl, combine one cup tomato sauce, garlic salt, onions, olives, cheese, and mashed beans.
2. Place 1/3 cup bean along center of each tortilla. Place the enchiladas in baking dish after it has been rolled.
3. Place the tomato sauce on top of the already filled tortillas. If desired, sprinkle with more cheese.
4. Bake for 20 minutes or until thoroughly heated.

41. *Bean Vegetable Casserole*

Yields: 4   Prep: 30 mins.   Cook: 1 hr. 30 mins.
Nutrition per Serving:
459 calories, 9 g fat, 76g carbs, 19 g fiber, 22 g protein

Ingredients:
- vegetable oil (3 tbs)
- onion, (1 large, chopped)
- celery, (2 stalks, chopped)
- green bell pepper (1 med, seeded and diced)
- tomatoes (2 med, seeded and diced)
- red kidney beans (2 cups, drained and rinsed)
- baby lima beans (2 1/4 cups, frozen and thawed)
- barley (1 cup)
- Italian parsley (2/3 cup, chopped)
- Salt (1/2 tsp)
- dried basil (1 tsp)
- cumin (1/2 tsp)
- boiling water (1 3/4 cups)

Directions:

1. Preheat oven to 350F degrees. In a non-stick pan, heat up the oil over medium heat. Add onion, celery, and green pepper.
2. Cook for 10 minutes or until vegetables soften. Stir the basil, lima beans, salt, barley, kidney beans, parsley, tomatoes, and cumin.
3. Take the mixture out of the pan and put it in a 3-quart casserole dish.
4. Ensure that the casserole dish has been sprayed with cooking spray that is not stick.
5. Add boiling water. Cover. Bake at 350 degrees for 1-1/2 hours.

42. Black Bean Quesadillas

Yields: 4   Prep: 10 mins.   Cook: 12 mins.
Nutrition per Serving:
203 calories, 1 g fat, 37 g carbs, 9 g fiber, 12 g protein

Ingredients:
- black beans (1 (28 oz) can, drained and rinsed)
- tomatoes (1/2 cup, seeded and chopped)
- cilantro (3 tbs, chopped)
- black olives (1/2 cup, pitted, halved)
- cumin (1/2 tsp)
- fat free Monterey Jack cheese (1/2 cup, shredded)
- fresh spinach leaves (2 cups, shredded)
- whole wheat tortillas (8 round)

Directions:
1. Preheat oven to 350 degrees. In a bowl, mash beans until smooth, but, slightly chunky.
2. Stir in tomato, cilantro and olives and cumin. Spread mixture evenly onto 4 tortillas. Sprinkle with cheese, and spinach.
3. Put the remaining tortillas on top. Bake the tortillas on a baking sheet that is not greased for 12 minutes.
4. Cut into wedges and serve.

43. Broccoli and Mushroom Rice

Yields: 4   Prep: 15 mins.   Cook: 25 mins.
Nutrition per Serving:
231 calories, 5 g fat, 41 g carbs,3 g fiber, 6 g protein

Ingredients:
- extra virgin olive oil (1 tbs)
- onion (1 medium, chopped)
- cloves garlic (2, minced)
- instant brown rice (1 cup)
- Portobello mushroom (8 oz., sliced)
- vegetable stock (3/4 cup)
- fresh broccoli florets (1 lb)
- salt (1/2 tsp)

Directions:
1. Preheat oven to 350F degrees. Set oil over medium heat in a nonstick pan to get hot.
2. Cook onions and garlic until soft, about 5 minutes. Stir in rice and mushrooms and cook 3-5 minutes or until mushrooms have released all of their juices.
3. Add the broth and bring to a boil. Reduce heat to medium-low and cover until liquid is absorbed (about 7 - 8 minutes).
4. Place broccoli in a casserole dish and sprinkle with salt and add 4 tbs. water.
5. Cover and cook at high power for 5 to 7 minutes or until tender. Place rice into a serving platter and top with broccoli.
6. Toss to combine and serve.

44. *Vegetable Curry*

Yields: 4   Prep: 10 mins.   Cook: 20 mins.
Nutrition per Serving:
298 calories, 28 g fat, 14 g carbs, 5 g fiber, 4 g protein

Ingredients:

- butternut squash (1 ½ lbs., seeded and chopped)
- olive oil (1 tbs)
- onion (1 small, finely sliced)
- curry powder (1 tbs, mild)
- coconut milk (1 2/3 cups)
- water (1 cup)
- fresh spinach (3 cups, chopped)
- butter beans (1 (14 oz) can, drained and rinsed)
- fresh cilantro (2 tbs, chopped)

Directions:

1. Add your squash with enough water to cover it in a saucepan then boil under tender. Drain and set aside.
2. Set a deep pot on medium heat with oil to get hot. Once hot, add in onions and cook until fragrant.
3. Add in your curry and stir for about 3 minutes being careful not to let it burn.
4. Add your water and coconut milk and allow to come to a boil.
5. Reduce heat, and simmer, without the cover, until thickened (about another 5 minutes).
6. Add in your remaining ingredients and stir until it's all heated through. Enjoy!

45.*Pork and Penne Pasta*

Yields: 4   Prep: 20 mins.   Cook: 30 mins.
Nutrition per Serving:
206 calories, 9 g fat, 24g carbs, 13 g fiber, 17 g protein

Ingredients:
- whole wheat penne pasta (1 lb.)
- ground Pork lean (1 lb)
- extra virgin olive oil (2 tbs)
- onion (1 small, chopped)
- garlic cloves (2, minced)
- can tomatoes (1 (15 oz), diced, seeded)
- green zucchini (2 cups sliced to 1/4 cubes)
- baby spinach (8 oz., fresh, chopped)
- low fat parmesan cheese (1 cup, grated)

Directions:
1. Bring a pot of water to a boil, ensure that the water is salted. Cook the pasta to an al dente consistency or according to package directions.
2. In a non-stick pan, cook the ground Pork over medium heat for 8 minutes or until it is browned, ensure to break up any large pieces in the pan.
3. Remove Pork and set aside. Discard drippings. Add in your oil on medium heat.

4. Cook onions and garlic for about 5 minutes or until soft. Add tomatoes and zucchini and continue cooking 5 minutes more.
5. Add spinach and cook until it just wilts, 2-3 minutes. Place the Pork back into the skillet and add 1/2 cup cheese; stir and heat through.
6. Plate your pasta then top with your meat mixture. Toss well and top evenly with cheese.

46. Chicken and Quinoa Pita

Yields: 4   Prep: 10 mins.   Cook: 0 mins.
Nutrition per Serving:
331 calories, 23 g fat, 5 g carbs, 2 g fiber, 26 g protein

Ingredients:
- fat free cream cheese (1 cup, softened)
- fat free mayonnaise (1 tbs)
- cooked chicken (2 cups, cubed)
- tomatoes (1 cup, seeded, sliced)
- Quinoa (1 (14 oz) can, cooked)
- romaine lettuce leaves (4)
- alfalfa sprouts (2 cups, rinsed, drained)
- whole wheat pita bread (4 round)

Directions:
1. In a bowl, combine mayonnaise and cream cheese until it is fully mixed.
2. Add chicken, tomatoes, Quinoa; mix well. Slice the pita bread to form a pocket.
3. Fill your pitas with lettuce and chicken. Top with alfalfa sprouts. Serve.

47. Chicken and Asparagus Pasta

Yields: 4   Prep: 10 mins.   Cook: 22 mins.
Nutrition per Serving:
168 calories, 10 g fat, 7g carbs, 3 g fiber, 13 g protein

Ingredients:
- whole wheat penne pasta (1 lb.)
- olive oil (2 tbs)
- chicken breast halves (3/4 lb, sliced into strips)
- poultry seasoning (1/2 tsp)
- cloves garlic (4, minced)
- asparagus (1 1/2 cup, frozen, cut into 1 inch)
- peas (1 cup, frozen, thawed)
- parmesan cheese (1/4 cup, grated)

Directions:
1. Set your salted water on to boil. Once boiling, add in your pasta then allow to cook until al dente (about 7 minutes) stirring to avoid sticking.
2. Set a non-stick pan on medium heat, add in a tablespoons of your oil then add in your chicken and season. Cook while stirring until golden.
3. Transfer your chicken from the pan to a plate and set aside.
4. Add in the rest of your oil, peas, garlic, and asparagus then cook while stirring until tender.
5. Add your chicken back to the pan on top of your pea mixture then let cook for another 2 minutes.
6. Serve your pasta and chicken topped with parmesan cheese.

48. Turkey Florentine

Yields: 4   Prep: 15 mins.   Cook: 18 mins.
Nutrition per Serving:
593 calories, 8 g fat, 11 g carbs, 4 g fiber, 12 g protein

Ingredients:

- olive oil (2 tbs)
- zucchinis (2 medium, seeded, thinly sliced)
- green onions (1/2 cups, sliced)
- turkey breast (2 cups, cubed)
- salt (1/2 tsp)
- thyme (1/2 tsp, ground)
- pimento (2 tbs, chopped)
- cooked long-grain rice (3 cups)
- fresh baby spinach (4 cups)
- low fat parmesan cheese (1/4 cup, freshly grated)

Directions:

1. In a non-stick pan, heat olive oil over moderate heat. Add zucchini, turkey, and onions, stir ever now and then for 5 to 10 minutes.
2. Add salt, thyme, pimento, rice and spinach. Cook and stir for another 6 - 8 minutes or until heated through and spinach wilts.
3. Remove from heat, transfer to large serving bowl, and stir in cheese. Serve.

49. Almond Salad

Yields: 1   Prep: 10 mins.   Cook: 0 mins.
Nutrition per Serving:
101 calories, 6 g fat, 10g carbs, 3 g fiber, 2 g protein

Ingredients:
- Blanched almonds (1½ cups, chopped)
- Olives (18)
- Celery (1½ cups, cut fine)
- Salad dressing (1 tbs)
- Lettuce

Directions:
1. Stone and chop the olives. Add the almonds and the celery.
2. Mix with salad dressing and serve on the lettuce.

50.Vegetarian Nuttolene Salad

Yields: 1   Prep: 10 mins.   Cook: 0 mins.
Nutrition per Serving:
55 calories, 0 g fat, 12 g carbs, 3 g fiber, 2 g protein

Ingredients:
- Nuttolene (¼ pound, Chopped)
- Celery (⅔ cup, Chopped)
- Protose (½ pound, Chopped)
- Onion (1 small teaspoonful, Grated)
- Lemons juice (2)
- Salt
- Mayonnaise (2 tablespoonfuls)

Directions:
1. Mix all the ingredients together, then add the mayonnaise dressing last. Serve

51. *Nutty Green Salad*

Yields: 4   Prep: 5 mins. Cook: 0 mins.
Nutrition per Serving:
252 calories, 2 g fat, 11 g carbs, 4 g fiber, 10 g protein

Ingredients:
- Walnut meats (1 cup)
- French peas (1 can)
- Mayonnaise (1 tbs)
- Lettuce (1 medium)

Directions:
1. Put the walnut meats in extreme hot water for fifteen minutes.
2. Remove the skins, then cut it into pieces. Set your peas to scald then set aside.
3. Drain the water from the peas, and let it get cold; then mix with the walnuts.
4. Add the mayonnaise dressing and mix thoroughly. Serve on lettuce.

52. *Asian Chicken Salad*

Yields: 1   Prep: 15 mins.   Cook: 0 mins.
<u>Nutrition per Serving:</u>
384 calories, 4 g fat, 68g carbs, 10 g fiber, 25 g protein

Ingredients:
- romaine lettuce (1 cup, chopped)
- carrot (1, shredded)
- celery (1, sliced thinly)
- red pepper (1/4 cup, seeded, sliced thinly)
- chicken breast (1/2 cup, cooked, cut into strips)
- mangos (1/4 cup, chopped)
- lime and ginger dressing (2 tbsp)

Directions:
1. Toss together all ingredients in a medium bowl until combined.
2. Serve alone or with whole wheat bread slices.

Conclusion

Thank you for sticking with me throughout this Diverticulitis Guide. I sincerely hope that the information, tips and recipes featured here were able to make your journey somewhat easier.

If you enjoyed what you read through, please take a moment to drop me a review on Amazon with your feedback. Let me know what worked for you or if any of the tips I shared was helpful to you in any way.

Cheers!

Printed in Great Britain
by Amazon

28896731R00089